Pocket Guide to Eczema and Contact Dermatitis

Pocket Guide to Eczema and Contact Dermatitis

Colin Holden

BSc, MD, FRCP
Consultant Dermatologist
Department of Dermatology
St Helier Hospital
Carshalton, Surrey

Lucy Ostlere

BSc, MRCP, MD
Consultant Dermatologist
St George's Hospital
London

b

**Blackwell
Science**

DISTRIBUTORS

  Marston Book Services Ltd
  PO Box 269
  Abingdon, Oxon OX14 4YN
  (Orders: Tel: 01235 465500
            Fax: 01235 465555)

USA
  Blackwell Science, Inc.
  Commerce Place
  350 Main Street
  Malden, MA 02148-5018
  (Orders: Tel: 800 759 6102
            781 388 8250
            Fax: 781 388 8255)

Canada
  Login Brothers Book Company
  324 Saulteaux Crescent
  Winnipeg, Manitoba R3J 3T2
  (Orders: Tel: 204 837 2987)

Australia
  Blackwell Science Pty Ltd
  54 University Street
  Carlton, Victoria 3053
  (Orders: Tel: 3 9347 0300
            Fax: 3 9347 5001)

A catalogue record for this title
is available from the British Library

ISBN 0-632-05663-0

Library of Congress
Cataloging-in-publication Data

Holden, Colin (Colin Arthur)
    Pocket guide to eczema and contact
    dermatitis/Colin Holden, Lucy Ostlere.
        p.   cm.
    ISBN 0-632-05663-0
    1. Eczema—Handbooks, manuals, etc.
    2. Contact dermatitis—Handbooks, manuals,
    etc. I. Ostlere, Lucy. II. Title.
    [DNLM: 1. Eczema—Handbooks.
    2. Dermantitis, Contact—Handbooks.
    WR 39 H726 2000]
    RL251.H65   2000
    616.5'21—dc21   00-023116

For further information on
Blackwell Science, visit our website:
www.blackwell-science.com

Contents

Preface

The eczemas account for approximately 10% of hospital referrals for skin conditions. The diseases affect all age groups and are increasing in incidence. They have a profound effect on quality of life and are a common cause of occupational disease.

Increasingly, management of eczema will be provided within the community, perhaps within dedicated nurse-led clinics.

There are many types of eczema and correct diagnosis is crucial to identify curable variants, to avoid mismanagement and to enable appropriate referral to hospital.

We hope that this short illustrated textbook will aid GPs and dermatology nurses in hospitals and the community to recognize eczema subtypes, to institute appropriate management and to pick out possible cases of contact allergy, which will allow appropriate referral for further diagnosis and management advice.

Colin Holden
Lucy Ostlere

Acknowledgements

Some of the information used for the preparation of the eczema section of this book was gathered in collaboration with Dr John Burton for Burton, J., & Holden, C.A., Eczema, lichenification and prurigo, Chapter 17, *Textbook of Dermatology*, 6th edn, 1998. Dr Holden gratefully acknowledges Dr Burton's collaboration in the updating of that information.

Section I: Eczema

1 Introduction

Eczema is the most common skin disease seen in general practice, accounting for approximately 20–30% of GP consultations about skin complaints. The terms 'eczema' and 'dermatitis' are generally regarded as synonymous, although some people consider dermatitis to imply an occupational or external cause as in contact dermatitis, whereas eczema implies an endogenous or genetic tendency.

The diagnosis, investigation and correct management of eczema depend on recognizing the features of eczematous change in the skin, determining the acuteness of the eczema and appreciating the pattern of the rash in order to establish the category of the patient's eczema (see Evaluation of eczema, page 8).

RECOGNIZING ECZEMA

The formal definition of eczema is a mixture of histological and clinical criteria.

Definition of eczema

Eczema is a syndrome of inflammatory skin reaction characterized histologically as spongiosis, with varying degrees of acanthosis and a superficial, perivascular, lymphohistiocytic infiltrate. The clinical features of eczema may include itching, redness and scaling, with clustered papulovesicles. A wide range of external and internal factors, acting singly or in combination, may induce the condition.

To expand on this, eczema is characterized by inflammation of the skin with epidermal changes. The hallmark of the epidermal change in eczema is oedema between the keratinocytes, causing them to separate. This is termed 'spongiosis'. In response to the inflammation, the epidermis thickens from either the oedema or the epidermal proliferation (acanthosis).

Clinically, this is seen in the skin of white people as an area of erythema, which is pink to red, and thickening of the epidermis with overlying crust

3

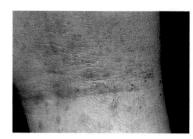

Fig 1.1 Subacute eczema.

and scale (Fig 1.1). Itching, burning and stinging are the usual symptoms. These symptoms provoke scratching and rubbing, which can give rise to secondary changes of excoriation and infection. In pigmented skin, erythema is more difficult to see and often skin thickening and the surface changes are more obvious in association with changes of hyper- or hypopigmentation.

ACUTE OR CHRONIC ECZEMA?

The appearance of eczema varies depending on the body site affected, the severity of the eruption and the duration of the rash.

Rapidly developing eczema or acute eczema is rare and usually more severe, with more prominent changes of epidermal oedema. The spongiosis is marked and the oedema increases to rupture the links between the keratinocytes, forming small fluid-filled cavities (vesicles) and eventually blisters (bullae). Eczema is derived from the Greek word meaning 'to boil' and these vesicles can be seen 'bubbling' at the surface in acute eczema. If these vesicles are pricked or scratched, they ooze serum (Fig 1.2).

In the much more common chronic eczema, spongiosis is much less intense and the reactive thickening of the epidermis (acanthosis) is the predominant feature. Clinically, this is seen as thickened darker skin with hyperkeratosis and increased skin markings, referred to as lichenification (Fig 1.3). Clearly, acute eczema can progress to chronic eczema and intermediate stages of subacute eczema can be seen. However, if chronic lichenified eczema shows marked crusting and weeping, secondary infection should always be suspected.

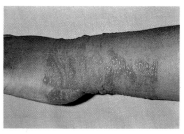
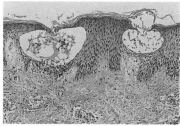

(a)   (b)

Fig 1.2 (a) Contact dermatitis to Elastoplast; (b) histology.

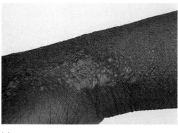
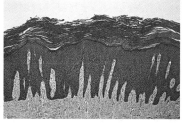

(a)   (b)

Fig 1.3 (a) Atopic dermatitis—lichenification; (b) histology.

Key points

The assessment of the acuteness of eczema is essential for its correct management because it determines the form or base in which topical treatments are applied.

Acute wet vesicular eczema requires treatment with antiseptic soaks (e.g. 1% aluminium acetate solution or 1/10 000 potassium permanganate solution), corticosteroid **lotions** or **creams**.

Dry chronic eczema requires greasy emollients and corticosteroid **ointments**.

CLASSIFICATION OF ECZEMA

Once the eczematous change in the skin is recognized, the specific diagnosis will usually be decided by the characteristic pattern or distribution

Table 1.1 The principal forms of eczema.

Exogenous	Endogenous
Irritant dermatitis	Atopic dermatitis
Allergic contact dermatitis	Seborrhoeic dermatitis
Photoallergic contact dermatitis	Lip-lick eczema
Infective dermatitis	Pityriasis alba
	Juvenile plantar dermatosis
	Pompholyx and hand eczema
	Lichen simplex
	Discoid eczema
	Asteatotic eczema
	Gravitational eczema

of the eruption. The principal forms of eczema are usually easily recognized by their distribution on the skin, and will allow their classification into exogenous and endogenous groups (Table 1.1). Exogenous eczema is related to clearly defined external trigger factors in which inherited tendencies play a minor role. The term 'endogenous eczema' implies that the eczematous condition is not caused by external environmental factors, but is mediated by genetic or constitutional processes originating within the body. Clearly, these boundaries are somewhat artificial and blurred, e.g. atopic dermatitis has a large genetic component but is aggravated by a wide range of environmental (exogenous) factors.

This point is most important because, although a diagnosis of endogenous eczema may be made, it is most important to consider curable or avoidable causes or aggravating factors before the condition is labelled as chronic eczema and purely symptomatic treatment prescribed. Thus, triggering of the dermatitis by infection (impetigo, tinea) is curable and irritants and allergens are avoidable.

SCABIES

Scabies must always be considered as a differential diagnosis for eczema. Characteristically, it produces a very itchy condition with severe night-time disturbance. The rash on the body is excoriated and eczematous but also spotty and patchy with a 'moth-eaten' appearance. There may be accentuation of the rash around the axillae, or involvement of the genitalia, and this should prompt thorough examination of the hands, wrists, ankles and feet for the tell-tale burrows. Remember that scabies affects all ages, and can be atypical in young infants and elderly people!

ECZEMA AND AGE

Certain patterns of eczema present more commonly in particular age groups. Most eczema in infants or young children is, or will develop into, atopic dermatitis. In atopic children, certain external factors can predispose to a specific presentation, e.g. lip-lick eczema or hand dermatitis, which are uncommon in non-atopic children. Pompholyx and hand dermatitis are most frequent in young adults and are less common in elderly people, whereas

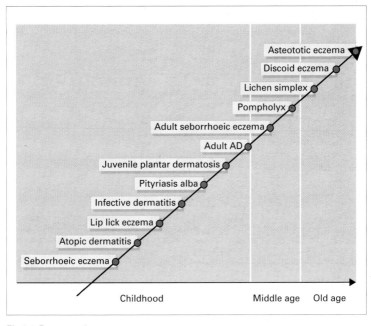

Fig 1.4 Eczema and age.

eczema associated with dry skin in winter, such as asteatotic eczema, is much more common in elderly people.

Figure 1.4 gives an approximate guide to the age of presentation of the different types of eczemas. In the first part of this book, the eczemas are discussed according to the age of presentation, starting with the eczemas of childhood, followed by the eczemas of early adult life and finally by eczema in later life. Irritant and allergic contact dermatitis can be a problem at all ages, although it is more common in adults than in young and elderly people, and is discussed separately in the second part of the book.

Evaluation of eczema

Morphology of the lesion
Is it eczematous—itchy, sore, red inflamed skin with epidermal change?
Is it acute—short history, wet oozy crusted vesicles, bullae?
Is it infected—clusters of erosions, pustules, golden crusting (consider swabs to identify herpes, *Staphylococcus aureus* and streptococci, and scrapes for tinea)?
Is it chronic—longer history, epidermal thickening, hyperkeratosis, increased skin markings, lichenification?

Age of onset
Child
Adult
Elderly person

Pattern of eruption
Symmetry often implies endogenous eczema
Flexural distribution in atopic dermatitis
Discoid lesions, etc

Is there an exogenous cause?
Irritant
Allergen
Infection

2 Childhood Atopic Dermatitis

DEFINITION
Atopic dermatitis (atopic eczema) usually begins in childhood as an itchy, chronic or relapsing dermatitis. It has an age-dependent distribution, appearing on the face and extensor surfaces in infants, but in the flexures of children and adolescents. More than 50% of children with atopic dermatitis have a personal or family history of asthma or hay fever.

DIAGNOSTIC CRITERIA
Recently, a UK working party developed a minimum set of diagnostic criteria validated for adult, paediatric and non-white ethnic groups (Table 2.1).

INCIDENCE
About 30% of the population are atopic. Recent reports of atopic dermatitis

Table 2.1 *Diagnostic criteria for atopic dermatitis.

Main condition	Three or more of:
An itchy skin condition (exclude scabies)	Onset below age of 2 years (not used if child is < 4)
	History of skin crease involvement (including cheeks in children < 10)
	History of a generally dry skin
	Personal history of other atopic disease (or history of any atopic disease in a first-degree relative in children < 4)
	Visible flexural dermatitis (or dermatitis of cheeks/forehead and outer limbs in children < 4)

The diagnosis of atopic dermatitis requires the patient to have an itchy skin condition plus three features from the right-hand column.
* From Williams HC, Burney PGJ, Pembroke AC et al. The UK working party's diagnostic criteria for atopic dermatitis III. Independent hospital validation, *Br J Dermatol* 1994; **131**: 406–16.

suggest a cumulative prevalence of 5–15% by the age of 7 years. There has been a two- to threefold rise in cases over the last 30 years, possibly as a result of environmental factors such as increasing levels of irritants and pollutants in homes. The annual cost to the UK economy has been estimated at £465 million.

PATHOGENESIS

Atopic dermatitis has a constitutional background. A gene predisposing to atopy has been found on chromosome 11q13 with weak linkage to maternal inheritance of atopic dermatitis.

Of people with atopic dermatitis, 80% show a raised serum immunoglobulin IgE and positive results to skin-prick tests for common allergens.

Biopsy of involved skin reveals chronic inflammation involving lymphocytes, mast cells, histiocytes and evidence of eosinophil degranulation. Atopic T lymphocytes release elevated levels of cytokines such as interleukin 4 (IL-4) after exposure, through a defective skin barrier, to aeroallergens or bacterial superantigens, e.g. staphylococcal exotoxins. Inflammatory mediators are produced more readily, possibly secondary to disordered intracellular control mechanisms.

Dry skin is a constant feature of atopic dermatitis. Even apparently normal skin shows defects of barrier function, increasing transepidermal water loss. Reduced ceramide lipids, which are essential to the formation of the skin's bilamellar, lipid membrane, water barrier, may explain this.

Thus, atopic dermatitis has the double handicap of an overactive atopic immune system and a defective cutaneous barrier to irritants and allergens.

Although these observations explain many of the features of the disease, the precise cause remains unknown.

CLINICAL FEATURES

The morphological features include the following.

1 Itching.
2 Macular erythema, papules or papulovesicles.
3 Eczematous areas with crusting.
4 Dry skin.
5 Secondary infection.

The peak age of onset is between 2 and 6 months. Itching often disturbs sleep and leads to extensive excoriation. The appearance of the disease varies with age.

INFANTILE PHASE

Characteristically, the rash starts on the cheeks (Fig 2.1), but it may occur anywhere. Generally, the nappy area is spared. Extensor involvement of the limbs may develop when the child begins to crawl. Initial lesions are oedematous, erythematous papules which may become confluent. They are often markedly excoriated with exudation and crusting. Intermittent morbilliform erythema may appear on the trunk when the dermatitis flares up. Secondary infection and lymphadenopathy often occur. More than 50% of babies gradually develop the flexural pattern of the childhood phase, although some are clear of the dermatitis by 18–24 months.

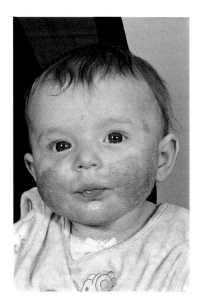

Fig 2.1
Childhood atopic dermatitis:
cheek rash.

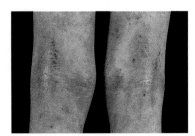

Fig 2.2 Lichenification of popliteal fossae.

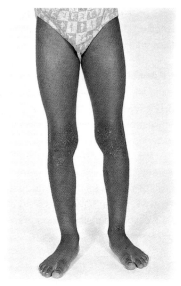

Fig 2.3 Extensor pattern of lichenification.

CHILDHOOD PHASE

The exudative oedematous lesions reduce and lichenification becomes predominant (Fig 2.2). Thickened excoriated skin, with increased skin markings, affects the antecubital and popliteal fossae, and the sides of the neck, wrists and ankles. Frequently, patchy and somewhat vesicular and lichenified eczema of the hand is seen and discoid patches of eczema are occasionally present on the limbs. In Afro-Caribbean, Asian and Chinese children, persistence of an extensor pattern with marked lichenification may be seen (Fig 2.3). Acute generalized or localized vesiculation suggests possible secondary bacterial or viral infection.

ADULT PHASE

This is essentially similar to the childhood phase. Pigment changes on the neck are common. Severely affected patients may show itchy facial erythema and flushing on a background of lichenification, which spreads to the upper chest, back and arms (see Chapter 5).

ASSOCIATED DISORDERS

Asthma or hay fever develops in approximately 50% of children with atopic dermatitis at about 2 and 8 years, respectively.

Dry skin occurs in most patients with atopic dermatitis. Up to 20% have ichthyosis vulgaris with associated keratosis pilaris and hyperlinear palms. However, keratosis pilaris can be seen without eczema as a dry follicular roughness on the outer aspects of the upper arms and thighs, with occasional lesions on the cheeks.

Contact urticaria is a common problem in atopic children. Contact with tomatoes, citrus fruits and Marmite may induce redness, swelling and itching of the perioral area or cheeks within minutes. This reaction may erroneously suggest that food allergy is the cause of the dermatitis. However, this reaction is caused by urticaria, not atopic dermatitis (Fig 2.4).

Atopic dermatitis is a cause of erythroderma or exfoliative dermatitis. Fortunately, this severe variety of the disease, which can occur at any age, is uncommon.

COMPLICATIONS

Quality of life

Atopic dermatitis severely affects the lives of both the patient and his or her family. Nocturnal scratching badly affects sleep, and in severe childhood cases can lead to behavioural difficulties that interfere with the functioning of the family.

Cutaneous infection

Staphylococcus aureus colonizes inflamed atopic skin. The bacteria may cause atopic dermatitis to flare up through activation of the immune system. In such a situation, antibiotic treatment may improve the dermatitis even in the absence of frank infection. Obvious infections, such as impetigo, are more common in atopic patients. Usually they are staphylococcal but may be caused by β-haemolytic streptococci. Nasal or groin carriage of staphylococci can sometimes be the source of recurrent cutaneous infections.

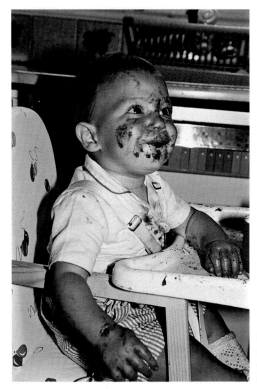

Fig 2.4
Food allergy: avoidance of
contact with irritant foods in
children can be difficult!

Viral infections

Patients with atopic dermatitis may develop generalized herpes simplex
infection or eczema herpeticum (Fig 2.5). Parents should be told about this
serious complication and warned that, if they have an active cold sore,
they should not kiss or cuddle children with atopic dermatitis. Eczema
herpeticum must be suspected in infected areas with tiny erosions or
crusts, and intravenous aciclovir therapy given, especially if there are
systemic symptoms of malaise, pyrexia, photophobia, etc.

Other viral infections, including warts and molluscum contagiosum, are
common and widespread in atopic patients.

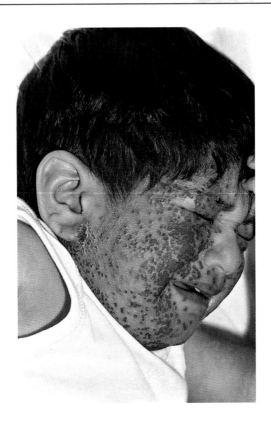

Fig 2.5
Eczema herpeticum.

Eczema is not a contraindication to immunization in children unless there has been an anaphylactic reaction to egg.

Growth retardation

About 10% of children with severe atopic dermatitis are small for their years. The evidence suggests that dermatitis itself may be the cause, rather than corticosteroid therapy, because intensive therapy can promote a growth spurt. Whatever the cause, children with severe disease should have their height and weight monitored.

Atopic cataract

Patients with severe atopic dermatitis occasionally develop bilateral atopic cataracts, usually between the ages of 15 and 30. They are at risk of developing corticosteroid-induced cataracts. There is also associated keratoconus.

DIFFERENTIAL DIAGNOSIS

In most instances, the diagnosis of atopic dermatitis is straightforward. However, scabies should always be excluded. In infants whose disease is unusually severe or where there are recurrent infections, failure to thrive, malabsorption or petechiae, immunodeficiency states should be considered.

OTHER CHILDHOOD ECZEMAS

For details of these, see Chapters 3 and 4.

INVESTIGATION

There is little need for investigation of the average patient with atopic dermatitis. IgE levels and radioallergosorbent tests (RASTs) are usually unhelpful for management and merely confirm the atopic nature of the individual. However, if a patient has a strong history of food allergy (usually causing abdominal symptoms or an urticarial eruption in association with eating the food), prick tests or RASTs are positive in only about 50% of cases. If the tests are negative, only 20% of children will have their eczema aggravated by the food. Therefore, the tests are a very inaccurate way of identifying suspect foods.

Bacterial swabs for culture should detect complications, such as antibiotic-resistant staphylococcal infection or the presence of β-haemolytic streptococci, or viral swabs should detect herpes simplex.

If immunodeficiency underlying the dermatitis is suspected, the appropriate referrals or investigations should be carried out.

MANAGEMENT

Management of atopic dermatitis is influenced by many factors, e.g. the patient's age, the extent of the disease, sites of involvement and the patient's home circumstances. Atopic dermatitis is a chronic, relapsing condition and must be treated accordingly.

Education

Education of the patient and parents of a child with atopic dermatitis is crucial and should be supported with written information. Useful information leaflets are available from the National Eczema Society (163 Eversholt Street, London NW1 1BU) and the British Association of Dermatologists (19 Fitzroy Square, London W1P 5HQ). Patients and their families must understand the condition and the expectations of therapy. Treatment can improve the disease, but no therapy can completely prevent relapse. Medical management should provide satisfactory control of the condition and minimize unwanted side effects of therapy.

Trigger factors

It is helpful to explain to patients that underlying their condition is an overly sensitive skin, in which inflammation can be triggered by a combination of a number of factors, with no single cause. Simple measures, such as turning down the temperature of central heating or wearing 100% cotton clothing, may make life more comfortable for the atopic patient.

Airborne allergens can aggravate atopic dermatitis and simple measures to reduce house-dust mite antigen may be advised, such as daily vacuuming and damp dusting of the bedroom. Similarly, animal dander irritates the skin, so the family should be discouraged from having pets.

Food allergy

Food allergies can be a trigger factor in 10% of children with eczema, but dietary therapy is controversial. Parents commonly institute a diet free of cows' milk without consultation; such diets are generally ineffective and inappropriate, and may cause malnutrition. Dietary therapy is a second-line treatment that requires careful supervision. Prick tests and RASTs are very inaccurate at predicting food allergy, and generally do not help disease management. A history of abdominal pain, diarrhoea or generalized urticaria associated with eating the suspect food may suggest an allergy, and trial of a diet avoiding that food is required for 6 weeks, during which the activity of the eczema is carefully monitored.

Contact urticaria to some foods is common; these foods can easily be avoided, but this does not improve the dermatitis.

Weaning
Introduce solids at 4–6 months, one food group at a time:
Milk-free baby rice
Puréed root vegetables
Puréed fruits (not citrus or berry)
Other vegetables
Cereals (wheat after 8 months)
Lamb and turkey (leave chicken and beef)
Fish after 10 months
Baby formula milk until 1 year
Leave eggs until after 1 year
Nuts after 4 years; chocolate only after 2 years

Table 2.2
Foods to delay during weaning of children with atopic dermatitis.

Breast-feeding should be encouraged, because of its general benefits, but the evidence that it modifies or prevents dermatitis is sparse. A mother who is unable to breast-feed and whose child develops atopic dermatitis should be reassured that she is not failing her child. The introduction of some foods should be delayed during weaning (Table 2.2) and peanuts should be avoided until after the age of 4 years.

Stress can aggravate atopic dermatitis. The severely affected child is a cause of stress for the whole family. The doctor's or nurse's role in offering simple reassurance and listening to family problems should not be underestimated.

FIRST-LINE THERAPY

Emollients

Dry skin is the major trigger in atopic dermatitis, and emollients should always be used when bathing. Bubble bath and household antiseptic additives should be avoided. Modern emollient bath additives are pleasant to use and may be used to target certain aspects of the disease, e.g.

those with lauramacrogols may help pruritus and antiseptic-containing oils may reduce infective episodes. Emollient creams should be used instead of soap. Moisturizing broken skin with emollients before bathing may be soothing and reduce stinging. Emollients should be applied immediately after bathing and can be reapplied as often as necessary throughout the day. The choice of emollient is very patient dependent. The author provides small quantities of several emollients from which the patient can select one. An emollient will not work if the patient does not use it! Large quantities (500 g/1 kg) should be prescribed thereafter. Each application may require 10 g or so depending on the age of the child.

Topical corticosteroids

Topical corticosteroids are used to treat inflamed areas. The reasons for using topical corticosteroids should be explained properly to the patient and parents, because the use of inappropriately weak or small amounts of topical corticosteroid is the main rectifiable problem after hospital referral. The strength of corticosteroid required varies with the situation. Generally, topical corticosteroids should be applied once or twice daily on to inflamed areas, using the weakest effective strength, until the inflammation settles. When the eczema returns, the treatment should be repeated. As a guide, the author uses 1% hydrocortisone ointment or other mildly potent corticosteroids in children aged under 1 year (and on the face in older patients). In children, the author aims not to use a stronger corticosteroid than the moderately potent group, which includes 0.05% clobetasone butyrate (Eumovate). However, severely thickened and lichenified areas, especially in older children and adults, require potent topical corticosteroid ointments, such as mometasone (Elocon), used in intermittent courses. Although creams may be used on weeping eczema for chronic conditions such as atopic dermatitis, ointments are more effective.

Topical corticosteroid and tar mixtures applied to lichenified skin can be soothing and help to reduce the strength of corticosteroid required. Combinations of antibiotics, such as Fucidin, and corticosteroids can be used to reduce staphylococcal contamination in flares of the dermatitis or infected skin. They must not be used for more than 2 weeks or resistance may develop.

Antibiotics

Flare-ups of dermatitis may be triggered by staphylococcal overgrowth, and a 5-day course of antibiotics such as flucloxacillin or erythromycin can help induce remission. Repeated infections can arise from staphylococcal carriage and Naseptin or Bactroban-Nasal ointment with an antiseptic bath oil (e.g. Oilatum Plus or Dermol 500) may be helpful in these circumstances.

Antihistamines

Itching is the major symptom of atopic dermatitis and no therapy specifically combats it. Sedative antihistamines, such as hydroxyzine or trimeprazine, can soothe nocturnal itching and have been widely prescribed for infants for many years. Non-sedating antihistamines have a minimal effect.

SECOND-LINE THERAPY

Most atopic dermatitis can be relieved by constant attention to the details above. If not, check for compliance, exclude antibiotic resistance and consider referral for second-line treatments.

Wet wrap technique

This helps the control of severe non-infected dermatitis in younger children. An inner layer of absorbent tubular bandage soaked in warm water is applied to the skin, which has been liberally covered in emollients (low-potency topical steroid is used in very severe cases). An outer dry layer of Tubifast bandage is applied. The dressings are left on overnight. Usually the parents can be taught the technique for use at home. Close supervision should be maintained if topical steroids are used, because suppression of the hypothalamic–pituitary axis can occur.

The strength of the topical steroid can be increased for 7–10 days. Localized areas of lichenification and excoriation on the limbs can be improved by nocturnal bandaging with cotton bandages impregnated with zinc oxide.

Children with severe dermatitis, and a strong suspicion of allergic triggers such as foods, should be referred to hospital for discussion of allergen management. The parents should be aware that this approach is not a cure, but helps only to modify the disease in a small proportion of children.

In severe cases, hospital admission for intensive topical treatment will settle the flare and allow the dermatitis to be better controlled at home.

THIRD-LINE THERAPY

Systemic treatments are usually initiated by consultant dermatologists. Gamolenic acid capsules (Epogam) reduce itch and dryness in a small proportion of patients with severe disease. Ultraviolet (UV) light therapy or psoralens plus UVA (PUVA) can help some adolescents with severe disease, particularly if there is evidence of growth retardation. Immunosuppressants, such as prednisolone, cyclosporin and azathioprine, are rarely required in children with atopic dermatitis.

Research is currently in progress with an immunosuppressive drug called tacrolimus, which may be used topically, and hence should be much safer for use in childhood.

Chinese herbal medicines are widely used by patients with atopic dermatitis. Although there are medical trials in adults and children that show a standardized decoction to be helpful, many patients are obtaining treatments from unlicensed and unrecognized Chinese centres. In these cases, it is impossible to be sure of the quality controls employed in the herbal decoctions. Even using the standardized formulation, some hepatotoxicity has been observed, and it is the toxicity of these treatments that are of concern.

PROGNOSIS

Roughly 75% of patients develop their dermatitis before 6 months of age and 80–90% by 5 years. Improvement occurs with age. About 50% of patients are clear of their dermatitis by the age of 13, but remission at puberty with recurrence in late adolescence or in the early 20s is not uncommon. However, few cases persist beyond the age of 30 years. Patients who have had atopic dermatitis need to be aware that their skin will continue to be sensitive throughout life.

CAREER ADVICE

Patients must realize that they have an in-built predisposition to irritant dermatitis. In particular, adolescents must be made aware that about 50% of occupational skin diseases occur in people with a background of atopy.

Young adults may decide on their future career having forgotten their childhood atopic dermatitis. Choosing a career that involves exposure to irritant chemicals or physical trauma may lead to the development of occupational dermatitis. It may then be too late to change career successfully.

3 Infantile Seborrhoeic Dermatitis

DEFINITION

Infantile seborrhoeic dermatitis is a non-itchy, red, scaling eruption with a predilection for the scalp, proximal flexures and nappy areas of infants.

AETIOLOGY

The condition appears to be unrelated to adult seborrhoeic dermatitis. Some dermatologists suggest that many cases turn out to be early-onset atopic dermatitis, or occasionally primary irritant nappy dermatitis with dissemination or infantile psoriasis.

In some cases, the yeast *Malassezia ovalis* has been found and the condition may respond to imidazole creams.

CLINICAL FEATURES

The rash most commonly starts at about 1 month of age. Usually it commences on the scalp with cradle cap and in the creases of the nappy area (Fig 3.1). The other proximal flexures and particularly the axillae become involved. If the face is involved, it has a tendency to favour the nasolabial creases and behind the ears.

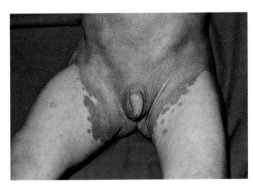

Fig 3.1
Seborrhoeic dermatitis in the nappy area.

Table 3.1 Comparison of the features of infantile seborrhoeic and atopic dermatitis.

Diagnostic factors	Seborrhoeic dermatitis	Atopic dermatitis
Age of onset	< 2 months	2–6 months
Pruritus	Uncommon	Common
Distribution of rash	Nappy area, axillae, scalp	Face, forearms, shins
Family history of atopy	30% of patients	> 50% of patients
IgE levels and RASTs to egg and milk	IgE normal, RASTs negative	IgE elevated, RASTs positive
Prognosis	Good: clears by 6 months of age; may progress to atopic dermatitis	Chronic and relapsing, associated with asthma and hay fever

RASTs, radio allergosorbent tests.

The rash has better-defined edges than typical atopic eczema with erythema and tiny vesicles. Greasy scales can develop which are particularly large and adherent on the scalp but smaller and drier in other areas.

The baby usually seems unconcerned by the eruption, which does not itch, and is happy, feeding and sleeping well.

The importance of the diagnosis is that the prognosis is good and the condition should resolve within a few months.

DIFFERENTIAL DIAGNOSIS

Atopic dermatitis is the main differential diagnosis. The main points of differentiation are shown in (Table 3.1). In practice, if the condition has not cleared within 3 months, atopic dermatitis is most likely.

4 Other Eczemas of Childhood

LIP-LICK ECZEMA

Definition
Lip-lick eczema is a moist or fissured eczema frequently spreading some distance around the mouth.

Aetiology
This condition most commonly occurs in atopic children, who often have typical atopic dermatitis elsewhere. As the name implies, constant chapping of the skin as a consequence of lip licking, lip smacking, thumb sucking or dribbling is the cause. The subsequent soreness of the skin provokes further licking and the condition becomes a habit. Occasionally, a true contact dermatitis to allergens, such as cinnamaldehyde in toothpaste, can be the cause.

In rare cases, contact urticaria to foodstuffs can be an aggravating factor. In this situation, the skin becomes red, swollen and itchy within minutes of contact with foods such as citrus fruits and juices and Marmite. Contact urticaria rapidly subsides within 20 minutes or so.

Clinical features
Red, sore, cracked eczema is seen frequently spreading some distance around the mouth (Fig 4.1). It may become secondarily infected and crusted.

Management
Management is to exclude any of the rare causes, usually on the history alone. The patient should be made aware of the role of habitual licking and chapping, and regular use of greasy protective moisturizers such as Vaseline advised, particularly overnight. If the skin is inflamed, the regular application of a 1% hydrocortisone ointment is usually most helpful. Recurrent infection is sometimes a consequence of staphylococcal carriage

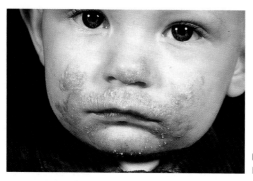

Fig 4.1
Lip-lick eczema.

in the nose. Although crusting around the nose may be seen, nasal swabs should be taken to identify silent carriage and appropriate oral antibiotics with BactrobanNasal or Naseptin ointment also prescribed.

INFECTIVE DERMATITIS

Definition
Infective dermatitis is diagnosed when a skin infection is a specific trigger of eczema rather than a complication of the dermatitis. It would be suspected when a child, who has never had dermatitis or whose eczema is in remission, suddenly has a flare-up of the condition with patches of eczema in association with skin infection. The eczema clears when the infection is treated.

Molluscum contagiosum
Molluscum contagiosum is the most common infection to trigger such attacks (Fig 4.2). Eczematous eruptions appear around clusters of molluscum, and sometimes a flexural dermatitis resembling atopic dermatitis can develop. When the molluscum infection clears or is treated, the eczema disappears. The eczematous reaction may represent immune recognition of the molluscum infection and herald its spontaneous resolution.

Clearly, this situation has to be distinguished from molluscum contagiosum complicating established atopic dermatitis, but it is a situation

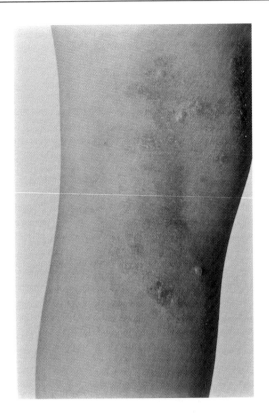

Fig 4.2
Molluscum contagiosum
causing a patch of eczema.

when active destruction of the molluscum lesions may be considered.
Mild corticosteroid creams can be considered if the eczema is distressing.

Infective dermatitis can also occur in association with tinea pedis. In this
situation, vesicular eczema on the feet may clear if the tinea is treated.

PITYRIASIS ALBA

Definition

This is a type of dermatitis that characteristically produces mildly red scaly
patches, which subside to leave areas of hypopigmentation.

Aetiology

Although more common in atopic individuals, pityriasis alba is not confined to atopic children.

Clinical features

Pityriasis alba occurs predominantly in children between the ages of 3 and 16. The individual lesion is a rounded, oval or irregular area, with fine bran-like scaling. Initially the erythema may be visible and there may even be minimal serious crusting at a few points on the surface of some of the plaques. However, the erythema may be very mild and subsides completely. Usually when seen by a physician, the patient shows only slight fine scaling and hypopigmentation. It is this loss of pigment that worries the patient, because in heavily pigmented skin it may be conspicuous and in lighter skins it may become so after suntanning (Fig 4.3).

The patches are often multiple, ranging in size from 0.5 to 2 cm in diameter, but may be larger. The lesions are often confined to the face and are most common around the mouth, chin and cheeks. In 20% of affected children, the neck, arms and shoulders are involved as well as the face. Less commonly, the face is spared and there are scattered lesions on the trunk and limbs. Most cases persist for some months and some may still show pale areas for a year or more after all scaling subsides. Recurrent crops of new lesions may develop at intervals. However, most children grow out of the condition eventually.

Diagnosis

The age incidence, the fine scaling and the distribution of the lesions usually suggest the diagnosis. Very pale patches, more common in the skin of Asian people, can lead to a misdiagnosis of vitiligo. However, in most cases the skin is hypopigmented and not depigmented as in vitiligo.

Treatment

It is most important to explain the diagnosis and emphasize that it is very rare for the hypopigmentation to be permanent. Although treatment is often disappointing, a bland emollient may reduce scaling. When the lesions are pink, a 1% hydrocortisone ointment may lessen the loss of pigment.

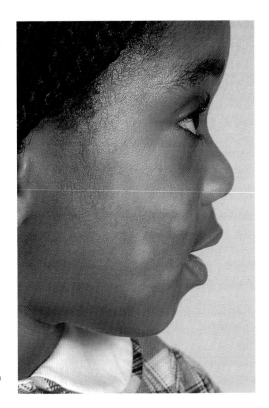

Fig 4.3
Pityriasis alba showing hypopigmented patches on the cheeks.

Routine application of sunblock to the whole face during the summer can reduce the contrast of the patches with the surrounding darker skin.

JUVENILE PLANTAR DERMATITIS

Definition

This condition is characterized by dry, fissured dermatitis of the plantar surface of the forefoot. It occurs almost exclusively in children aged 3–14 years and was first recognized as a condition in 1968.

Aetiology

The precise cause of the condition is unknown. Although many children are atopic, few have active atopic dermatitis in other sites. One theory is that increased use of synthetic materials in the composition of children's socks and shoes in the last 30 years or so may be responsible for the emergence of this disease. Synthetic materials are generally less porous than the natural materials that they have replaced. The feet are thus subjected to hot, humid conditions that encourage mild maceration, particularly in children who may wear trainer shoes throughout their waking hours. Many of the affected children are keen on sports, which suggests that friction and enhanced sweating may be playing some part.

Clinical features

Very few cases have been reported in adults or infants. There is a slight preponderance of male patients. The presenting features are redness and pain in the plantar surface of the forefoot, which assumes a glazed and cracked appearance (Fig 4.4). The condition is most severe on the ball of the foot and toe pads, tending to spare the non-weight-bearing instep. The toe clefts are normal, and this helps to distinguish the condition from tinea pedis. The symmetry of the lesions is a striking feature. Occasionally, the disease can affect the dorsum of the feet or the hands, with painful and fissured palms or fingertips. This is more likely in children with active atopic dermatitis. The most severe symptom is pain from deep cracks that can develop on weight-bearing surfaces.

Diagnosis

This is a clinical diagnosis, although skin scrapings to exclude tinea pedis should be taken if there is doubt about the diagnosis. Allergy to components of footwear is rare but, if suspected, referral for patch testing may be required.

Treatment

Most cases will clear spontaneously in due course, but the condition may persist until adolescence. Parents and children are usually advised to change from non-porous footwear to 100% cotton socks and leather shoes or sandals, although the evidence that it helps is minimal. In severe cases

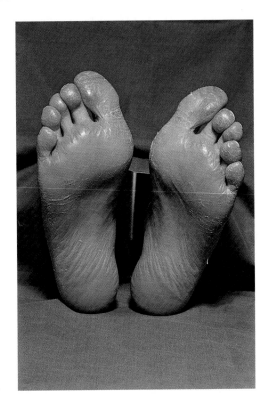

Fig 4.4
Juvenile plantar dermatitis.

with painful cracking, Micropore tape applied across the split as a splint can soothe. Emollients applied regularly, such as 50% white soft paraffin and liquid paraffin, may help. Sometimes they need to be applied overnight under occlusion by Clingfilm wrapped around the foot and covered by a sock. Others, including urea preparations, Lassar's paste, white soft paraffin or tar, may help but no single preparation works in all cases.

5 Adult Atopic Dermatitis

The majority of atopic dermatitis is seen in children and most cases clear by adulthood, with 50% of patients being clear of the condition by the age of 13. Nevertheless, many cases of adult atopic dermatitis are seen. It is unusual for a typical case of atopic dermatitis to start for the first time in adult life, and fewer than 2% of all cases start after the age of 20. However, atopic dermatitis may go into remission at puberty and then flare up in early adult life, particularly if the patient has entered an occupation with a high exposure to irritants.

CLINICAL PATTERNS

1 Frequently the picture is similar to that in later childhood, with lichenification, especially of the flexures, periorbital area (Fig 5.1) and hands. Localized patches of atopic dermatitis can occur on the nipples, especially in adolescent and young women. Involvement of the vermilion of the lips and the adjacent skin is commonly an atopic manifestation (Fig 5.2). Follicular lichenified papules are rather characteristic in pigmented skin.

2 A distribution on the face, upper arms and back may correlate with the areas of maximal thermal sweating or sensitivity to *Malassezia ovalis*. In chronic adult atopic dermatitis, reticulate pigmentation on the neck may be seen (Fig 5.3).

3 Photosensitivity is not uncommon in adults with atopic dermatitis. This may cause exacerbation of the dermatitis on sun-exposed sites and a seasonal variation, depending on the wavelength of light to which the patient is sensitive.

4 A patchy vesicular hand dermatitis and a more diffuse chronic lichenified eczema of the hands are frequently found in cases of adult atopic dermatitis. Atopic dermatitis is often a contributory factor in many cases of what usually has to be called constitutional hand eczema (see page 41). A previous history of atopic dermatitis is also a significant factor in the development of occupational dermatitis.

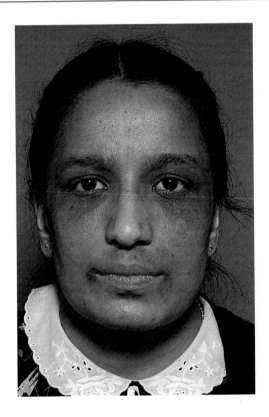

Fig 5.1
Atopic blepharitis.

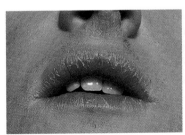

Fig 5.2 Atopic dermatitis: facial rash.

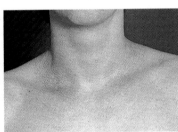

Fig 5.3 Atopic neck.

CATARACT

This occurs in more severe adolescent and adult cases, but overall it is rare. It is associated with atopic dermatitis, apparently independent of steroid use, rather than with other atopic diseases. The peak incidence is between the ages of 15 and 25.

DIFFERENTIAL DIAGNOSIS AND INVESTIGATION

Adult atopic dermatitis is usually associated with current, or a history of, other atopic diseases. However, a flare-up of eczema in adult life when the disease has been in remission should prompt a search for new trigger factors. Enquiries should be made about occupational or lifestyle exposure to irritants or contact allergens and, if these are suspected, the patient should be referred to a dermatologist for patch testing. Nickel allergy can sometimes present with a flexural dermatitis mimicking that of typical atopic dermatitis. Allergies to medicaments or moisturizer should also be considered if a life-long atopic dermatitis has an exacerbation.

The sudden onset of a generalized, itchy, eczematous rash should always raise the suspicion of scabies, and appropriate history and examination undertaken.

Food allergy as a cause of dermatitis is seen in less than 1% of atopic adults. However, contact urticaria to natural latex protein, e.g. rubber gloves, is on the increase. This can cross-react with certain foods such as bananas and kiwi fruit (see page 103).

MANAGEMENT

The principles of the management of adults are the same as those for children (see page 16). However, often more potent topical steroids may be required, depending on the body site affected.

Patients with the head and neck pattern of atopic dermatitis may benefit from a trial of itraconazole tablets (100 mg daily for 21 days) with a hydrocortisone/imidazole (e.g. Daktacort) ointment topically. In a proportion of patients sensitive to malassezia yeasts, this can be helpful.

The management of photosensitive eczema is specialized and such patients should be referred to a dermatology unit.

Patients who do not respond to the first- and second-line approaches as described for childhood sufferers should also be referred for consideration of more powerful therapies.

These include phototherapy with UVB or UVA or a combination of the two. Photochemotherapy (PUVA) can help atopic dermatitis. Unfortunately, the doses and frequency of radiation may have to be greater than in psoriasis, with a correspondingly increased risk of skin cancer. X-ray irradiation has been used in occasional adult cases where there is gross lichenification restricted to localized areas.

A number of systemic therapies are available for recalcitrant cases. Limited effectiveness or concerns over toxicity often restrict their usefulness. Cyclosporin has been shown to be effective in control of adult atopic dermatitis in low dosage. Renal toxicity is the limiting factor.

Oral corticosteroids have a limited but definite role in helping patients with very severe atopic dermatitis over flare-ups of their disease. Long-term treatment often requires doses that will lead to typical side effects.

Chinese herbal medicines have been subjected to medical trials, and decoctions of a standard formulation appear helpful in adults. Concern has been expressed about their hepatotoxicity.

Several other drugs may be effective in atopic dermatitis such as azathioprine, interferon-γ and topical tacrolimus ointment.

PROGNOSIS

Even in adults with persistent atopic dermatitis, improvement can be achieved by appropriate attention to lifestyle and good topical treatment. Systemic therapies may have to be continued for some years but most patients' eczema will gradually diminish and few will have typical flexural eczema after the age of 30.

However, atopic hand dermatitis, occupationally related problems and photosensitive eczema can be very persistent.

6 Adult Seborrhoeic Dermatitis

DEFINITION

This is a chronic dermatitis with a distinctive morphology (red, inflamed, well-defined lesions with greasy-looking scales). Adult seborrhoeic dermatitis has a distinctive distribution, appearing in areas with rich supplies of sebaceous glands, namely the scalp (associated with dandruff), face and upper trunk.

Seborrhoeic dermatitis affects 3–5% of young adults, although mild degrees of dandruff are much more common. It is common in HIV infection. The condition is rare before puberty, and the peak age of onset lies between 18 and 40.

AETIOLOGY

The yeast *Malassezia furfur* (syn. *Pityrosporum oviculare*) is increased in the scaly epidermis of dandruff and seborrhoeic dermatitis, and is widely accepted as the causative agent. This may be why seborrhoeic dermatitis is common in immunodeficiency. The disease responds to several different antifungals which seem to have as their only common feature an anti-malassezial effect.

Maturation of the sebaceous glands may be a permissive factor for the development of seborrhoeic dermatitis. Many young adults with the condition appear to have a greasy skin.

CLINICAL PATTERNS

There are several clinical variants of seborrhoeic dermatitis, which occur in various combinations and degrees of severity.

Scalp

Dandruff is usually the earliest manifestation. At a later stage, perifollicular redness and scaling extend to form sharply marginated patches, which may remain discrete or coalesce over the greater part of the scalp and extend to

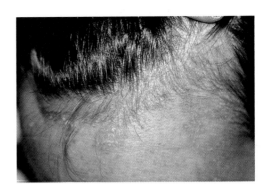

Fig 6.1
Seborrhoeic dermatitis.

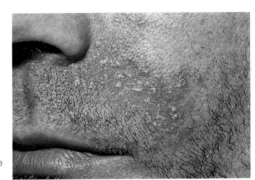

Fig 6.2
Seborrhoeic dermatitis of the
nasolabial folds.

the forehead as the 'corona seborrhoeica' (Fig 6.1). In chronic cases, there
may be some hair loss that recovers as the inflammation is suppressed.
Redness and greasy scaling often develop behind the ears, with a crusted
fissure in the fold. Persistent otitis externa may accompany seborrhoeic
dermatitis in other sites or may occur alone.

Face

Facial seborrhoeic dermatitis involves the medial side of the eyebrows,
between the eyebrows and the nasolabial folds (Fig 6.2), usually in
association with involvement of the scalp.

Blepharitis

Blepharitis is common; in this condition, the margins of the lids are red and covered by small white scales and yellow crusts. Exposure to sunlight produces a temporary exacerbation, followed by improvement as a tan develops.

Young women sometimes have paranasal erythema associated with a tendency to flushing. It is not always clear whether this is rosacea or mild seborrhoeic dermatitis, but over-treatment with strong topical corticosteroids may convert this into a variant of rosacea called perioral dermatitis.

Trunk

The most common truncal rash is seen in men on the front of the chest (Fig 6.3) and in the interscapular region. The initial lesion is a red–brown follicular papule, covered by a greasy scale. Confluence of the follicular papules gives rise to multiple circinate patches, with larger greasy scales at their margin.

Flexures

In the proximal flexures, seborrhoeic dermatitis presents as an intertrigo with diffuse, sharply marginated erythema and greasy scaling. A crusted fissure develops in the folds and, with sweating, secondary infection and inappropriate treatment, a weeping dermatitis may extend far beyond them.

Seborrhoeic folliculitis can be seen in association with seborrhoeic dermatitis. The condition most commonly affects men. The rash comprises erythematous follicular papules and follicular pustules. Lesions occur mainly on the upper trunk and shoulders, and are usually itchy. The absence of comedones, cysts and scars distinguishes it from acne vulgaris. All patterns show a tendency to chronicity and to recurrence. Occasionally, seborrhoeic dermatitis may become generalized, resulting in erythroderma.

DIAGNOSIS

Nowadays, it is important to consider the possibility of HIV infection in any patient with severe seborrhoeic dermatitis. Psoriasis confined to the scalp may be confused with seborrhoeic dermatitis. Psoriasis is usually palpably

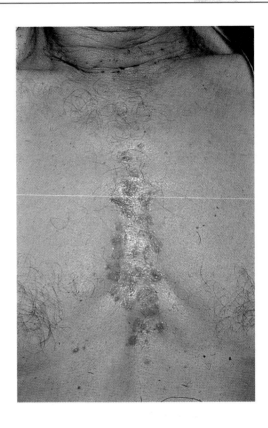

Fig 6.3
Seborrhoeic dermatitis of
sternal area of chest.

thickened, brighter pink in colour, with a silvery scale. The rest of the body
must be examined, especially the nails, and there may be a family history of
psoriasis. In the flexures, mycological examination of scrapings from the
advancing margin can exclude ringworm infections and candidiasis. Wood's
light examination will reveal the coral pink fluorescence of erythrasma.
Acute flexural dermatitis may suggest allergic sensitization to a chemical
in clothing, and patch tests may be needed. The brown scaly lesions of
pityriasis versicolor are easily distinguished. Microscopy of scrapings
quickly establishes the diagnosis.

TREATMENT

Although the eruption can be suppressed, the condition may require regular treatment for many years. Dandruff is treated by the regular use of medicated shampoos against malassezia yeasts, including selenium sulphide, pyrithione zinc, ketoconazole and various tar shampoos. For severe dandruff with persistent scaling or crusting, 5% salicylic acid ointment may be useful. If secondary infection is suspected, swabs may reveal staphylococcal infection and appropriate antibiotics should be prescribed orally.

Acute seborrhoeic dermatitis on the face and trunk is sensitive to mild steroid creams with or without a combined imidazole. Ketoconazole cream (Nizoral) 2% is suitable therapy for long-term use. In many situations, the acute inflammatory changes are suppressed by mild topical corticosteroid creams or steroid and imidazole cream combinations, which can be changed to ketoconazole cream for long-term control. Lithium succinate (Efalith) 5% ointment has also been shown to be effective.

For unresponsive cases, itraconazole (100 mg daily for up to 21 days) is effective. Subsequent once-weekly use of ketoconazole shampoo as a shower gel may help prevent relapse of truncal rashes and folliculitis.

Referral to hospital may be sensible in severe cases to exclude rarer differential diagnoses and make hospital-based treatments such as UVB phototherapy available to the patient.

7 Pompholyx and Hand Eczema

DEFINITION

The term 'hand eczema' implies dermatitis largely confined to the hands, with only minor involvement of other areas. When the hands are involved only coincidentally within a widespread eczema, it is preferable to speak of hand involvement. Up to 30% of occupational medical practice centres on hand eczema, and contact allergic and irritant dermatitis should always be considered (see page 73) before diagnosing endogenous hand eczema.

Most cases of hand eczema are multifactorial. This not only makes treatment difficult, but it can also cause considerable problems in medicolegal cases (e.g. occupational dermatitis in which negligence is alleged against an employer).

Atopy, naturally dry skin, superadded contact allergic or irritant dermatitis, or even the effect of rubbing or scratching, may all obscure the original cause. Even the daily mild trauma of normal life and climatic influences may play some part.

ENDOGENOUS CAUSES

Atopy is the most common endogenous cause of hand eczema. Hand eczema is more common in people with a history of atopic dermatitis. The hands are the most common site of adult atopic dermatitis. In some patients, the hands alone are involved. Indeed, hand eczema in an adolescent or young adult when he or she becomes exposed to school, hobby or occupational irritants may be the first atopic manifestation. The eruption is often patchy and always very irritable. Lichenification is evident at an early stage, and pompholyx may be present. Atopy also predisposes to a discoid pattern of hand eczema in young adults. Atopic hand eczema probably has the worst prognosis of all types of hand eczema.

POMPHOLYX

This is vesicular eczema of the palms and soles.

Definition

Pompholyx is an eczema of the palms and soles, in which oedema fluid forms visible vesicles or bullae. The thick epidermis in these sites causes blisters to become large before they burst. Pompholyx on the palms is called cheiropompholyx and, on the soles, podopompholyx.

Aetiology

In most cases no exogenous cause is found. The role of the sweat glands is disputed. Although the distribution of the lesions matches that of palmoplantar sweating, and the condition is worse in hot weather, hyperhidrosis is not a constant feature. A personal and family history of atopy occurs in half of all patients with pompholyx.

Primary irritants can provoke pompholyx, e.g. metal workers exposed to soluble oils. Occasionally, contact allergens cause an asymmetrical, palmar, pompholyx-like reaction.

Inflammatory fungal infection, usually on the feet, can provoke eczema of the palms. Previously, this was diagnosed frequently but now is regarded as rare. In some patients, recurrences can be related convincingly to stressful episodes, but in many others there is no such correlation. It should be remembered that pompholyx itself causes stress, particularly if there are financial problems caused by loss of work. Aspirin ingestion, oral contraceptives and cigarette smoking increase the risk of pompholyx.

Clinical features (Fig 7.1)

Pompholyx occurs at any age but it is rare in those under 10 years, and more common before the age of 40. A pompholyx attack is characterized by the sudden onset of crops of 'frog-spawn'-like groups of clear vesicles. There is no erythema, but a sensation of heat and prickling of the palms may precede attacks. Vesicles may coalesce to form large bullae, especially on the feet. Severe itching may precede the eruption of vesicles. The attack subsides spontaneously and resolves with desquamation in 2–3 weeks. Recurrent attacks in this period cause continuation of symptoms in a minority of cases. In mild cases, only the sides of the fingers may be affected, but in a typical case the vesicles develop symmetrically on the palms and/or soles. In 80% of patients only the hands are involved.

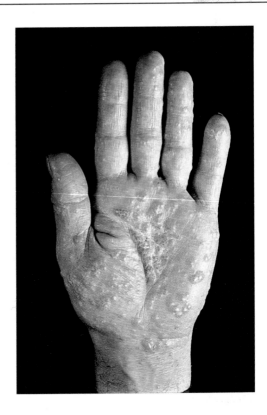

Fig 7.1
Pompholyx.

Unilateral or asymmetrical patterns should alert the physician to look for contact or infective causes of the eruption.

Secondary infection with pustule formation and lymphangitis is common and may complicate each attack in certain patients. After recurrent attacks spreading to the dorsum of the fingers, the nails may develop dystrophic changes, irregular transverse ridging and pitting, thickening and discoloration.

Recurrences are usual. They occur at regular intervals for months or years, or at long irregular intervals. Pompholyx is more common in warm weather, and in some patients attacks occur each summer.

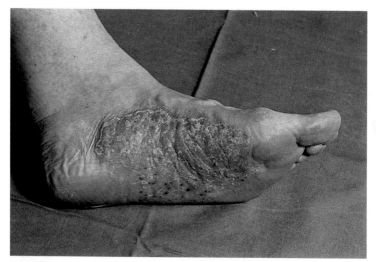

Fig 7.2 Pustular psoriasis.

Diagnosis

An asymmetrical area of scaling and vesiculation of the palm or sole should suggest dermatophytosis and scrapings should be examined for fungus. If the erythema is limited to one or two interdigital clefts, is asymmetrical or involves the dorsal skin to any extent, contact dermatitis must be excluded by a careful history and referral for patch testing.

In palmar–plantar pustular psoriasis, there are usually no clear vesicles. The pustules are sterile and leave characteristic brown marks as they resolve (Fig 7.2). Occasionally, bacterial infection of pompholyx occurs with pustule formation, but in these cases the lesions tend to be painful, with surrounding erythema, and culture of the pus yields the causative organism.

Treatment

Any cause for the eruption should be eliminated. In the acute phase, the hands or feet should be soaked three times a day in either potassium permanganate solution (diluted 1:10 000—it will stain the skin, nails, clothes, etc., so warn the patient!) or Burrow's solution (aluminium acetate 1%). Large bullae may be aspirated using a sterile syringe. Systemic antibiotics are required if bacterial infection develops. Staphylococcal infection is most likely, but occasionally streptococci are found and penicillin with flucloxacillin or erythromycin is usually effective. As the eruption subsides, the soaks should be discontinued and potent topical corticosteroid creams applied. Steroid creams containing antibiotics or antiseptics such as fusidic acid (Fucidin H) and Clcoquinol (Vioform-Hydrocortisone), respectively, may be more effective. In severe cases a course of oral steroids may be justified.

For chronic pompholyx in the dry hyperkeratotic phase, tar preparations such as 2–5% crude coal tar may be used, or a potent steroid ointment preparation may be combined with a coal tar solution.

HYPERKERATOTIC PALMAR ECZEMA

This distinct form of hand eczema is characterized by highly irritable, scaly, fissured, hyperkeratotic patches on the palms and palmar surfaces of the fingers (Fig 7.3).

The aetiology is unknown. Patch tests are usually negative, and the incidence of atopy and psoriasis is no greater than in a normal control

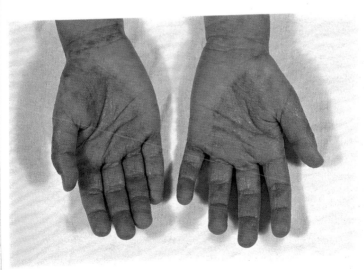

Fig 7.3 Hyperkeratolic palmar eczema.

population. However, if the condition is not responding to treatment, hospital referral for exclusion of contact allergy should be considered.

Differential diagnosis

Hyperkeratotic hand eczema can be confused with psoriasis. Most dermatologists have confidently diagnosed hand eczema in patients who have later developed typical psoriasis. Even biopsy may not be diagnostic. In most cases of psoriasis on the hands, however, the silvery nature of the scale, involvement of the knuckles, sharply demarcated 'scalloped' edges to the erythema along the borders of the hands and fingers, and the relative absence of pruritus are helpful pointers. The family history of psoriasis and the presence of nail pits in the absence of proximal nail fold lesions are also suggestive.

Tinea can also be missed (Fig 7.4). Unilateral scaling of the palm suggests a possible infection with *Trichophyton rubrum*.

The whole skin should be examined in any case of hand eczema in which the diagnosis is in doubt. There may, for example, be evidence of nickel allergy or tinea pedis, or small patches of psoriasis of which the patient is

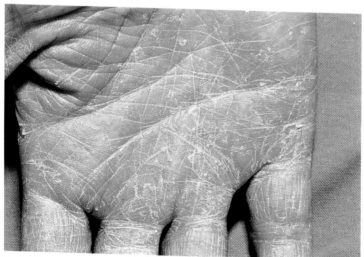

Fig 7.4 Tinea manium.

unaware. Hand dermatitis significantly affecting a patient should be referred to a dermatologist to exclude contact allergy before chronic endogenous hand eczema is diagnosed.

TREATMENT OF CHRONIC HAND ECZEMA

Once contact allergy has been excluded, the same general principles of treatment apply as for chronic eczema elsewhere. Three useful measures are as follows.

1 Avoidance of irritants.
2 Frequent application of emollients.
3 Sparing use of topical steroids.

Avoidance of irritants is difficult because they are so ubiquitous. Education of the patient alerting them to the possible dangers is most important and advice leaflets can be very helpful (see the Lucy Ostlere advice leaflet in Table 7.1).

Table 7.1 Advice Leaflet.

Hand dermatitis

To speed healing and prevent relapse of your dermatitis the following are suggested:

Handwashing: use lukewarm water and a soap substitute, e.g. Diprobase, aqueous cream or emulsifying ointment. Avoid all soaps

Irritants: avoid direct contact with irritants, e.g. detergents, cleaning agents and solvents. If possible avoid direct contact with shampoos and use plastic gloves when washing hair

Rings: avoid wearing rings in situations where moisture or irritants, e.g. soap, may get trapped under the ring.

Gloves: avoid rubber gloves (as some people are allergic to these) and use plastic or PVC gloves (found in, for example, Sainsburys or Boots). Cotton gloves may be worn under the plastic or PVC gloves for comfort. Avoid wearing gloves for more than 20 minutes at a time

In cold weather, wear gloves when outdoors

The resistance of the skin is lowered for up to 6 months after the eczema has healed so continue to follow these instructions.

Cleanliness helps, but too much soap and water can be harmful. A wide variety of soap substitutes is now available. Brief exposure to soap followed by immediate application of an emollient may be beneficial by removing bacteria and debris.

Gloves provide the best protection. Holed gloves are worse than no gloves at all, but thick gloves may make it impossible to perform a particular task. Rubber gloves generally give good protection for housework. For patients with rubber allergy, polyvinyl chloride (PVC) household gloves are available. If sweating makes the condition worse, cotton gloves worn beneath the protective gloves may help. Thin leather gloves should also be used for dry work to prevent soiling and trauma, especially for gardening in cold dry air.

Emollients should be rubbed frequently into the skin, and jars should be left near sinks, etc. so that they are readily available. The choice of emollient varies with the patient. Some like greasy preparations such as an emulsifying ointment, whereas others prefer more cosmetically acceptable creams such as an aqueous cream. Numerous commercial preparations are now available. Some topical preparations sold over the pharmacy counter as antipruritics or emollients can contain irritants such as alcohol or propylene glycol, and patients should use the creams that the physician recommends.

Topical steroids are used in the weakest effective strength. However, potent steroids are usually required and these occasionally cause atrophy. Although the palms are thick, the epidermis can be rendered thin and fragile by long-term use of potent topical steroids. This is not a major problem in hyperkeratotic eczema.

A systemic antibiotic may be needed for bacterial infection, and the use of a combined steroid–antiseptic or antibiotic combination preparation may be more effective.

In unresponsive cases, use of a potent steroid under occlusion may be considered. The steroid is applied at bedtime, under polythene gloves worn overnight. Although an effective treatment, it greatly increases the risk of atrophy and secondary bacterial infection, and should be discontinued as soon as possible.

Painful fissures of the fingertips are a problem. The main treatment is to keep the keratin soft by the use of greasy preparations, often under polythene occlusion at night. Fissures, once formed, are slow to heal, but they can sometimes be rendered less painful by splinting them with Micropore tape.

If hand eczema does not respond to topical steroid therapy, the diagnosis should be reviewed, particularly with regard to the possibility of tinea. The patient should be asked again about exposure to irritants or allergens, and referred to the dermatologist.

Tar pastes may help chronic unresponsive cases. Generally speaking, messier preparations such as 5% crude coal tar tend to be more effective than more cosmetically pleasant preparations. Salicylic acid ointment 2–5% may improve hyperkeratosis and persistent scaling. Various combinations of tar, steroids and salicylic acid may be tried.

More potent therapies are available but these are usually given under hospital supervision. Oral psoralen chemotherapy (PUVA) and UVB therapy have proved useful for recalcitrant hand eczema. Radiotherapy can help stubborn hand eczema.

Acitretin is used for hyperkeratotic eczema, but there is a high incidence of side effects and cyclosporin has been reported to be useful in recalcitrant cases.

8 Lichen Simplex

DEFINITION

Lichen simplex is a patch of thickened skin caused by scratching. There is an accentuation of the surface markings so that the affected skin surface resembles tree bark.

Although lichenification may be secondary to a pruritic dermatosis, the term 'lichen simplex' is used where there is no known predisposing skin disorder. There appears to be well-marked racial variation in the capacity of the skin to lichenify, and the high incidence of lichenification in black and Asian people has often been emphasized.

In the predisposed subject emotional tensions play an important role in favouring the development of lichenification and ensuring its perpetuation.

CLINICAL FEATURES

In lichen simplex pruritus is the predominant symptom and is often out of proportion to the appearance. It may develop in paroxysms of great intensity. Scratching tends to give great satisfaction initially, but is continued with violence until the skin is sore and there is then a refractory period of some hours until the itch recurs. During the early stages the skin is reddened and slightly oedematous, and the normal markings are exaggerated. The redness and oedema subside and the central area becomes scaly and thickened and sometimes pigmented. Surrounding this central plaque is a zone of lichenoid papules and, beyond this, an indefinite zone of slight thickening and pigmentation merges with normal skin.

The peak incidence of lichen simplex is between the ages of 30 and 50. There can be single and multiple lesions, usually at sites that are conveniently reached, such as the nape of the neck, the lower legs and ankles (Fig 8.1), the sides of the neck, the scalp, the upper thighs, the vulva, pubis or scrotum, and the extensor forearms.

Lichen simplex of the nape of the neck, lichen nuchae, is almost entirely confined to women. The plaque may be a small area around the midline of the nape or may extend into the scalp. 'Notalgia paraesthetica' is a small patch of itchy lichenified skin at the inferior tip of the scapula.

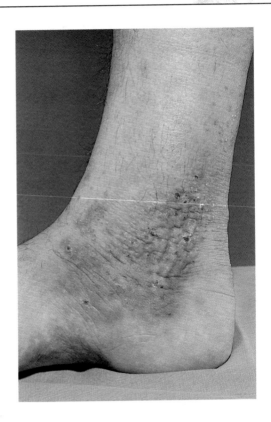

Fig 8.1
Lichen simplex.

DIAGNOSIS

The diagnosis is not usually difficult—lichen planus and psoriasis have to be excluded and typical lesions should be sought in other sites. Sometimes biopsy of the patch may be helpful, but a patient with psoriasis can occasionally develop lichen simplex, which combines the histological features of both conditions.

Once the diagnosis of lichenification has been established, its causation must be carefully investigated. Symmetrical lesions in particular should suggest secondary lichenification of a contact dermatitis (see page 69).

TREATMENT

The nature of lichen simplex, and the need to break the scratching habit, must be explained to the patient, as should the association with stressful events and tension. In most cases, a potent steroid ointment is the treatment of choice. A useful trick for resistant cases (on appropriate body sites) is to apply a potent steroid scalp lotion, allow it to dry and cover with a sheet of Granuflex. This can be left for up to a week, and is repeated once weekly for up to a month.

Modest improvement has also been shown with 5% doxepin cream. Circumscribed chronic lesions are often most effectively treated by dermal infiltration with triamcinolone (10 mg/ml).

9 Asteatotic Eczema

DEFINITION

Asteatotic eczema is associated with a decrease in skin surface lipid and characterized clinically by a cracked 'dry river bed' appearance. The synonyms are winter eczema and eczema craquele.

AETIOLOGY

The condition is thought to be caused by a decrease in skin surface lipid. This can be caused by the following:

- a naturally dry skin and a lifelong tendency to chapping;
- a further reduction in lipid with age, illness, malnutrition or hormonal decline;
- chapping and degreasing from industrial or domestic cleansers or solvents;
- low environmental humidity or dry cold winds.

A patient will often ascribe the onset to an event or change in life that is quite trivial, e.g. a particularly cold dry winter. Years of contact with industrial degreasing agents may be tolerated until, usually in the patient's 50s or 60s, a small additional hazard precipitates a disabling eczema.

Diuretics and myxoedema may provoke asteatotic eczema in elderly people.

CLINICAL FEATURES

The condition occurs particularly on the legs, arms and hands. The skin is dry and slightly scaly. The surface of the backs of the hands is marked in a criss-cross fashion, as though the continuity and flexibility of the keratin had been disturbed. The finger pulps are dry and cracked.

On the legs, the pattern of superficial markings is more marked and deeper (Fig 9.1) (a 'crazy-paving' pattern or 'dry river bed' appearance). The borders of the cracks become erythematous and slightly raised, and frank eczematous changes finally develop.

Irritation in this form of eczema is often intense and worsens with changes of temperature, particularly on undressing at night.

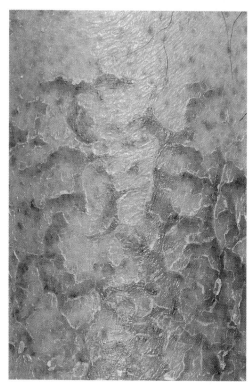

Fig 9.1
Asteatotic eczema.

The condition can persist for months, relapsing each winter and clearing in the summer, but eventually becoming permanent. Discoid eczema can also occur on this background, although the relationship between the two conditions is uncertain.

TREATMENT

The patient's immediate environment may need to be adjusted. Central heating should be humidified where possible and abrupt temperature changes should be avoided. Wool is usually poorly tolerated and possibly damages by irritation. Patients are often more comfortable wearing thin cotton clothing against the skin. Baths without oils are best limited and should not be hot. Emollients should be used after bathing and every day. The greasier moisturizing preparations are generally most helpful. Lotions should be avoided.

Moderate topical corticosteroid ointments containing fusidic acid (Fucidin) or an antiseptic should be applied to the inflamed areas. Corticosteroids contained in a urea base are very appropriate in this situation because urea encourages hydration.

This is one of the forms of eczema in which soaps and detergent cleansers can be seen by the physician and felt by the patient to be deleterious, and the regular use of soap substitutes in the autumn and winter may help prevent relapses.

10   Discoid Eczema

DEFINITION

Discoid eczema is characterized by a single, non-specific, morphological feature, namely circular or oval plaques of eczema with a clearly demarcated edge.

AETIOLOGY

In most cases the cause is unknown; it can occur in both atopic and non-atopic individuals and contact allergy is uncommon.

Local physical or chemical trauma plays a part in some cases, and discoid eczema sometimes develops at the site of an old injury or scar. Dry skin resulting from low environmental humidity is sometimes associated with discoid eczema. Emotional stress may play a role in some cases, but it is unlikely to be the primary cause. An association between excessive alcohol and discoid eczema has been reported.

Heavy colonization of the lesions by staphylococci may increase their severity, even in the absence of clinical evidence of infection.

CLINICAL FEATURES

Morphology

The diagnostic lesion of discoid eczema is a coin-shaped plaque of closely set, thin-walled vesicles on an erythematous base. In the acute phase the lesions are dull-red, oozy, crusted and highly irritable (Fig 10.1). They progress towards a less vesicular and scalier stage, often with central clearing, and peripheral extension, causing ring-shaped or annular lesions. As they fade, they leave dry scaly patches. Between 10 days and several months later, secondary lesions occur, often symmetrically on the opposite side of the body and then to other limbs or the trunk. It is very characteristic of this disease that dormant patches may become active again, particularly if treatment is discontinued prematurely.

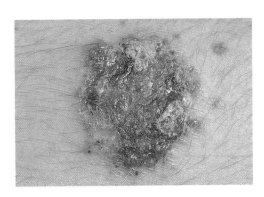

Fig 10.1
Discoid eczema.

CLINICAL PATTERNS

Discoid eczema of the limbs and trunk

Discoid eczema affecting the limbs and trunk is the most common, occurring in managerial or professional classes, and in elderly people with dry skin exacerbated by low humidity, such as central heating. The initial patch usually occurs on the lower leg and secondary lesions spread to the other leg (Fig 10.2), the arms and often the trunk. The lesions may become increasingly oedematous and crusted, possibly because of secondary infection. Extension then becomes rapid and, in severe cases, much of the trunk and limbs will be involved. Scattered papulovesicles may be interspersed with large and small plaques.

All forms of discoid eczema are chronic, with partial remission during which plaques tend to clear in their centres. Most forms tend to relapse and are at their worst during the colder months of the year.

Discoid eczema of the hands and forearms

Discoid eczema of the hands affects the dorsal surface of the hands or the backs or sides of individual fingers. It often occurs as a single plaque at the site of a burn or a local chemical or irritant reaction. Secondary lesions may occur on the hands, fingers or forearms. It is a not uncommon form of irritant occupational dermatitis, but may also occur in housewives or secretaries in whom the provoking factors are less clear. An atopic history

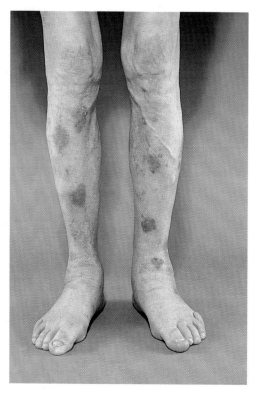

Fig 10.2
Secondary lesions of discoid eczema.

appears to be more frequent in young women with discoid hand eczema than in other forms of the disease.

'Dry' discoid eczema

'Dry' discoid eczema is uncommon, consisting of multiple dry scaly round or oval discs on the arms or legs (Fig 10.3), but also with scattered microvesicles on an erythematous base on the palms and soles. Itching is minimal, and the condition persists for several years, with fluctuation or remission. The condition is notably resistant to treatment.

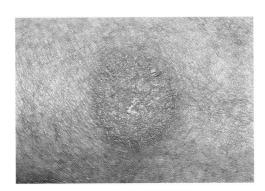

Fig 10.3
'Dry' discoid eczema.

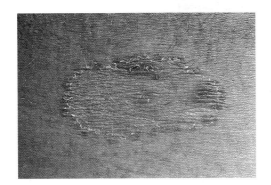

Fig 10.4
Tinea corporis (ringworm).

DIAGNOSIS

Discoid eczema may simulate ringworm but, even when the lesion of discoid eczema clears in the centre, the edge is broader, more vesicular and more vivid in colour than those caused by trichophyton infection, where scaling of the edge is a more conspicuous feature (Fig 10.4). Scrapings should be examined for the presence of ringworm fungi.

In psoriasis, the lesions are dry, the scaling is more prominent and the irritation milder. The ring-shaped lesion of granuloma annulare is not scaly (Fig 10.5).

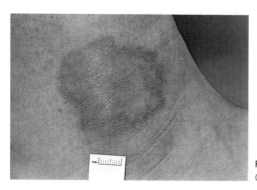

Fig 10.5
Granuloma annulare.

TREATMENT

Usually a potent topical steroid is needed, perhaps with added clioquinol or fusidic acid (Fucidin). Dilute forms are relatively ineffective. Coal tar pastes or ointments may be added in the less acute, drier stages. Emollients and bath oils to moisturize the skin may help to prevent relapses. Oral antibiotics such as erythromycin can help in severe exudative cases. In severe cases, oral steroids may be required. General considerations such as the avoidance of irritants apply, as with other forms of eczema.

11 Erythroderma

'Erythroderma' is the term applied to any inflammatory skin disease that affects more than about 90% of the body surface. Often there is continuing exfoliation of scale, and the term 'exfoliative dermatitis' is sometimes used synonymously. Eczema is one of the main causes of erythroderma (Table 11.1).

Although generalization of eczema occurs most frequently in people in their 50s and 60s, atopic erythroderma may occur at any age. Exacerbation of existing lesions usually precedes the generalization, which follows the usual pattern. Pruritus is often intense. Erythroderma is a serious disease and is particularly dangerous in elderly people. Death can occasionally result.

Chronic generalized erythroderma is associated with profound metabolic disturbances. The blood flow through the skin increases markedly and this can result in high-output cardiac failure, especially in elderly patients. The increased skin perfusion may lead to hypothermia.

Fluid lost by transpiration is much increased and the loss of exfoliated scale may reach 9 g/m² of body surface or more each day. Hypoalbuminaemia is common and diminished immune responses may lead to infection.

Common	Rare
Eczema	Hereditary disorders
Psoriasis	Lichen planus
Drug reactions	Crusted scabies
Cutaneous lymphoma	Pemphigus

Table 11.1
Causes of erythroderma.

TREATMENT

Treatment in hospital is advisable because some cases may develop serious general medical problems. In these cases, the protein and electrolyte balance, the circulatory status and the body temperature require continual surveillance. The environmental temperature must be carefully regulated. Cooling and overheating must both be avoided by the use of extra blankets or fans. Systemic complications should be monitored for and treated as required. The possibility that the erythroderma is the result of a drug reaction should be considered in every case, and all non-essential drugs should be withdrawn.

The cutaneous inflammation should be treated in the first instance with soothing emollient creams or a mild topical steroid. Most patients will improve over a week or two on this regimen, during which time the diagnosis of the underlying condition will probably be established. Many dermatologists prefer to avoid systemic steroids if possible, because of the dangers of fluid retention, secondary infection, diabetes, etc., but in severe persistent cases they may become necessary. Antibiotics may be required to control secondary infection.

Section II: Contact Dermatitis

12   Introduction

Around 2% of the population are affected by contact dermatitis. Skin problems account for up to a third of all occupational disorders and the majority of these are contact dermatitis. There are two types of contact dermatitis—irritant and allergic—often referred to as irritant dermatitis and contact dermatitis, respectively.

IRRITANT DERMATITIS

This is the result of damage to the skin by irritants and typically affects the hands. Common irritants are water, soaps and detergents. Substances used in industry such as cement, cutting oils and acids are also important. All individuals will develop irritant dermatitis if the irritant is strong enough and in contact with the skin for long enough, although individual susceptibility does differ.

CONTACT DERMATITIS

This is the result of a delayed-type hypersensitivity reaction. The allergen penetrates the skin and attaches to the Langerhans cells in the epidermis which migrate, via the lymphatics, to the regional lymph nodes. There the allergen encounters T lymphocytes, resulting in allergen-specific T cells which proliferate and circulate. It takes around 7–10 days before there are enough allergen-specific T cells to produce contact dermatitis. After sensitization, dermatitis can develop within 2–3 days of contact with the allergen.

It is not always possible to distinguish allergic contact dermatitis from irritant dermatitis or endogenous eczema by appearance alone, and patch testing is an essential tool for diagnosis. Testing is important because if the cause is identified and avoided, the patient's dermatitis may be cured. Even short cutaneous contact in a sensitized individual may result in a flare of the eczema. Treatment of contact dermatitis in the acute stage is the same as that for endogenous eczema, i.e. application of emollients and appropriate topical steroids.

13   When to Suspect Contact Dermatitis

The results of patch testing cannot always be predicted, although in some instances the history is fairly reliable. For example, patients who describe developing dermatitis with non-silver/non-gold jewellery will usually be allergic to nickel and/or cobalt. Studies have shown that, if the dermatitis is caused by only one allergen, the results can be predicted in around 70% of cases. However, if the cause of the dermatitis is multifactorial, the results will be predictable in only around half the cases. The group of allergens that is most difficult to detect is medicaments, such as wool alcohols and neomycin, the latter being predicted correctly in only 8% of patients in one study.

Hands are constantly being exposed to irritants and potential allergens, and not surprisingly they are the most common site of contact dermatitis. When a patient presents with hand dermatitis, one needs to consider whether the dermatitis is endogenous, irritant or allergic, or whether it is a combination of these factors (see page 41). Even if endogenous or irritant dermatitis is suspected, patch testing should still be carried out because it is not clinically possible to rule out contact allergy. The second most common site of contact dermatitis is the face, followed by those sites that are exposed to chronic medicament usage, namely the lower legs (venous ulcers and stasis eczema), anogenital region (chronic pruritic conditions) and ears (chronic otitis externa). Table 13.1 shows the groups of patients in whom patch testing should be considered.

When patch testing should be considered:
Other skin diseases, e.g. psoriasis that is worse with treatment
Persistent anogenital dermatoses, otitis externa and periorbital dermatitis
Chronic hand and foot dermatitis
Chronic occupational dermatitis

Table 13.1
Indications for patch testing.

WHEN IS PATCH TESTING NOT APPROPRIATE?

Patch testing is important because detecting an otherwise unsuspected contact allergen and avoiding it may result in a patient's dermatitis being cured. However, there are occasions when patch testing is not appropriate, as shown in Table 13.2.

A common misconception that patients have is that their dermatitis is caused/exacerbated by foods, and not infrequently they will attend the

Table 13.2
Examples of when patch testing is not appropriate.

When patch testing is not appropriate:
Typical atopic dermatitis or mild dermatitis that responds to treatment
Patients requesting allergy testing to foods
Diagnosis is not dermatitis, e.g. psoriasis

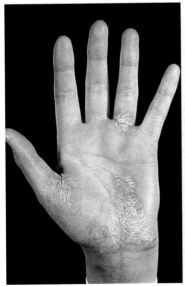

Fig 13.1 Psoriasis of the palm.

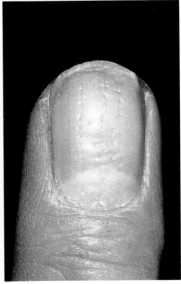

Fig 13.2 The nail, showing pitting typical of psoriasis.

dermatology clinic expecting to be 'allergy tested to foods'. Evidence suggests that, particularly in adults, 'food allergy' rarely plays a role in the development of dermatitis (see page 107). Well-recognized reactions to foods are acute generalized urticaria and contact urticaria, and testing for these types of allergic reactions is discussed in Chapter 17.

Psoriasis is sometimes mistaken for hand dermatitis (Fig 13.1). This should always be considered and other sites, namely nails (Fig 13.2), elbows, knees, scalp, umbilicus and natal cleft, examined. In most patients with psoriasis, patch testing is not helpful. However, patch testing should be considered if there is an eczematous element to the psoriasis, or if the topical treatment appears to be making the psoriasis worse, or when a coexistent contact allergy is suspected.

14 Clinical Patterns of Contact Dermatitis

Although contact dermatitis may occur on any part of the skin, certain sites are more frequently affected. Tables 14.1 and 14.2 show some of the areas where contact dermatitis is most commonly seen and list some of the common allergens and their sources.

FACE

Allergens can affect the face by direct contact or indirectly by airborne or hand-to-face exposure. In addition, close contact with another individual

Table 14.1 Products that can cause dermatitis of the face, ears and neck and their potential allergens.

Site	Allergens	Source
Face	*Preservatives*, e.g. Cl + Me-isothiazolinone	Cosmetics and creams
	Fragrance Wool alcohols	
	Toluenesulfonamide formaldehyde resin	Nail varnish
	Airborne contacts, e.g. Sesquiterpene lactone Phosphorous sesquisulphide Fragrances	Compositae plants Some matches Perfumed sprays
	PPD	Hair dyes
Eyelids	Parabens Colophonium	Mascara/eye shadow
	Benzalkonium chloride	Eye-drops, contact lens solution
Ears	Nickel Neomycin	Earrings Ear-drops

Cl + Me-isothiazolinone, chloro-methyl-isothiazolinone; PPD, *P*-phenylenediamine.

Table 14.2 Products that can cause dermatitis of the body and their potential allergens.

Area of the body	Allergen	Source
Periaxilla, antecubital fossa and other sites	PPD	Clothing dyes
Axilla	Fragrance, formaldehyde	Deodorants
Waistline	Rubber allergens, nickel	Elastic in underwear, jeans studs
Genital area	Rubber allergens Fragrance Parabens, neomycin, benzocaine, Balsam of Peru	Condoms/diaphragms Perfumed soaps, etc. OTC and prescribed creams
Hands	Rubber allergens Thiopropanol *S*-oxide Diallyldisulphide Formaldehyde	Rubber gloves Onion Garlic
Feet	Chromate; rubber allergens; PTBP resin; PPD	Leather Soles of shoes Glues of shoes Dyes in socks and shoes
Varicose eczema	Rubber allergens; parabens; wool alcohols, neomycin; quinolone mix	Elasticated stockings; medicated stockings and creams; topical preparations

PPD, *P*-phenylenediamine; OTC, over the counter; PTBP, 4-*tert*-butylphenol formaldehyde resin.

(consort dermatitis) may result in contact allergy. Cosmetics are the most common source of contact dermatitis as a result of direct contact. Patients develop a dermatitis that can be intermittent or continuous depending on the frequency of cosmetic application. Common allergens in cosmetics include fragrances, wool alcohols and various preservatives, e.g. parabens, chloro-methyl-isothiazolinone and quaternium 15 (see Fig 14.1). Products that are labelled 'Hypoallergenic' or 'For sensitive skin' still contain preservatives. Since 1997, all cosmetics and skin care products must be fully labelled with the INCI (International Names of Cosmetic Ingredients).

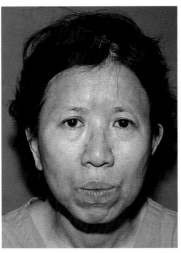 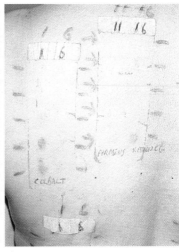

(a)   (b)

Fig 14.1 (a) A patient who presented with a facial dermatitis. (b) The patient's patch test results show positive reactions to parabens (methylparaben, propylparaben, ethylparaben, butylparaben) and Kathon CG (methylchloroisothiazoline (and) methylisothiazolinone). The patient was advised to avoid these preservatives in creams and cosmetics and given the INCI name (as shown in brackets). She also coincidentally had a positive reaction to cobalt (see page 82), which was not relevant to her facial dermatitis (the dark dot above cobalt is the PPD [*p*-phenylenediamine dye] patch test).

It is therefore important that patients with positive patch tests are given the INCI name of their allergens.

A patient with facial dermatitis may not think of nail varnish as the cause. Nail varnish allergy usually produces an asymmetrical dermatitis affecting the eyelids, face and neck (Fig 14.2). The most common allergen is toluenesulfonamide formaldehyde resin.

The scalp is particularly resistant to contact allergy, so hair dyes generally produce dermatitis of the hairline, eyelids, ears, neck and hands.

Airborne allergens produce a dermatitis in exposed sites. Causes of airborne dermatitis include plants, e.g. the Compositae group of plants (see Fig 15.10, Chapter 15, page 89). Sunlight can also play a role, giving these patients a light-aggravated dermatitis which will be worse in the summer.

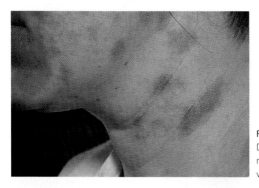

Fig 14.2
Dermatitis of the face and
neck secondary to nail
varnish allergy.

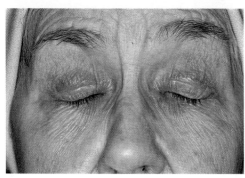

Fig 14.3
Periorbital dermatitis
caused by a preservative
in eye-drops.

Red-headed matches containing phosphorus sesquisulphide classically
produce an asymmetrical facial dermatitis.

EYELIDS

Make-up can cause eyelid dermatitis by irritant or allergic reactions.
Allergens include preservatives, e.g. parabens, and colophonium (may be
found in mascara and eye shadow). Eyelid dermatitis may also result from
indirect transfer of substances from either the hand or airborne dermatitis.
Allergy to contact lens solutions and prescribed eye-drops may result in a
periorbital dermatitis (Fig 14.3). In addition, periorbital dermatitis is a feature
of atopic dermatitis (particularly in adults) and 'sympathetic dermatitis'
associated with a contact dermatitis from another site. As the skin around
the eye is loosely bound, dermatitis is often associated with oedema.

EARS

The most common cause of ear-lobe dermatitis is nickel from earrings, and patients with nickel allergy should wear solid silver or gold jewellery (see page 81). Postauricular dermatitis may be secondary to plastic or metal allergy from spectacles or plastic hearing aids. Contact dermatitis is also well recognized in the ear canal, and an inflamed and excoriated external auditory canal is particularly susceptible to sensitization. Common allergens include neomycin, benzocaine and parabens from topical medicaments. Endogenous causes of erythema and scaling in the ear, such as seborrhoeic dermatitis and psoriasis, should also be considered.

AXILLA

An irritant dermatitis from deodorants and hair removal is well recognized, as is an allergic dermatitis caused by perfumes and preservatives (e.g. formaldehyde) in deodorants. Clothing dermatitis, most commonly resulting from clothing dyes, typically affects the anterior and posterior folds of the axilla with sparing of the apex.

HANDS

The three main causes of hand dermatitis are:

1 endogenous
2 irritant
3 allergic.

However, in many cases there is some overlap and all three may be contributing factors. Important points in the history are shown in Table 14.3.

Table 14.3 Important points in the history of a hand dermatitis patient.

Is the patient atopic or is there a family history of atopy? (see page 9)
Are their hands exposed to irritants, e.g. decorators, cleaners?
Are their hands exposed to excessive water and washing, e.g. bar staff, mothers of young children, nurses?
Are their hands exposed to common allergens either at home or at work, e.g. hairdressers, builders, contact with glues and rubber gloves?

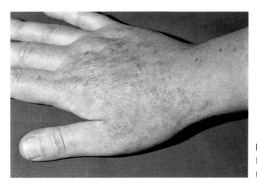

Fig 14.4
Irritant dermatitis in a nurse
(patch tests were negative).

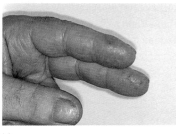

(a)

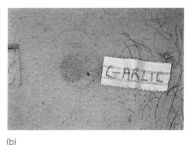

(b)

Fig 14.5 (a) Dermatitis on the thumb and forefinger caused by garlic allergy. (b) Patch test results show a positive reaction to garlic.

Clinically, it is not possible to distinguish reliably between the different causes of hand dermatitis. Both contact and irritant dermatitis may predominantly affect the dorsum of the hand (Fig 14.4). It is, therefore, important that all patients with persistent hand dermatitis are patch tested to see whether a contact allergy (and therefore an avoidable cause) is present.

Any allergen can cause hand dermatitis. Table 14.4 shows some of the well-recognized causes of contact allergy in the hands.

Treatment of hand dermatitis is shown on page 47. If a contact allergy is identified, this must be avoided. As with all patients with contact dermatitis, they should be aware that the allergy is life-long and only a short exposure to the allergen can result in a recurrence of the dermatitis.

Table 14.4 Allergens that may cause hand dermatitis, with examples of their source and clinical features.

Allergen	Suspect	Common clinical features and site involved
Rubber allergens; thiurams, MBT, mercapto mix	Gloves	May extend up to mid forearm with sharp cut-off
Chromate	Cement; leather gloves	
PPD	Hair dyes	
Nickel	Jewellery, watches	Localized to site of ring/watch etc.
Primin	Primulas	Streaks of vesicular dermatitis
Epoxy resin	Glues	Fingertips
Colophony	Paper	Palmar aspect of middle and index fingertips and thumbs
Thiopropanol *S*-oxide	Onion; thiopropanol S-oxide	Palmar aspect, fingers and thumb
Diallyldisulphide	Garlic	Palmar aspect of middle and index fingertips and thumbs
Topical preparations		
Preservatives (e.g. parabens)	Eurax, E45	
Wool alcohols	Alpha Keri Bath Oil, Oilatum bath emollients; creams, e.g. Sudocrem, Synalar ointment	
Cetyl steryl alcohol	Creams, e.g. Diprobase, Unguentum Merck	
Tixocortol pivalate	Hydrocortisone	
Neomycin	Cicatrin, Dermovate-NN and Betnovate-N	

MBT, mercaptobenzothiazole; PPD, *P*-phenylenediamine.

Table 14.5 Allergens seen in foot dermatitis and their sources.

Allergen	Parts of shoe
Chromate	Uppers, insoles
Rubber allergens (MBT and thiurams)	Soles
PTBP resin	Glue used for shoe lining and insole

Rarer causes of shoe dermatitis include colophony (used in glues), dyes and nickel. MBT, mercaptobenzothiazole; PTBP, 4-*tert*-butylphenol formaldehyde.

FEET

Contact dermatitis affecting the feet is usually symmetrical and tends to occur at the site of shoe contact with sparing of the instep, the flexural aspect of the toes and the interdigital spaces. A shoe dermatitis may result in autosensitization and 'sympathetic dermatitis' affecting the hands. Patients may also be patch tested to pieces of the potentially offending shoe. Table 14.5 shows the common allergens seen in foot dermatitis.

Patients with foot dermatitis who are found to be allergic to one of the above need to avoid the allergen for life. Wearing shoes that contain the allergen even for a short period of time can result in an exacerbation of dermatitis. Clarks make a range of leather, rubber or 4-*tert*-butylphenol formaldehyde (PTBP) resin-free shoes and other shops sell leather-free shoes (see Appendix). Unfortunately, despite careful avoidance, the prognosis for shoe dermatitis is poor. There are a number of possible reasons for this: first, some allergens may be difficult to avoid; and, second, patients may find it difficult to wear only their hypoallergenic shoes. In addition, in some patients there may be an element of endogenous eczema.

ANOGENITAL AREA

Allergic contact dermatitis in the anogenital area commonly results from applied medicaments. In women, allergic contact dermatitis is more likely when there is involvement of the perianal area as well as the vulva. Figure 14.6 shows a patient with a long-standing pruritic inflammatory dermatosis (lichen sclerosus) who has relevant positive patch tests. Another important

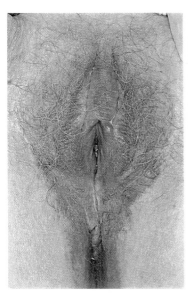

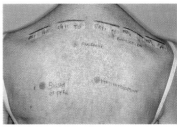

(b)

(a)

Fig 14.6 (a) A patient with lichen sclerosus (note the white atrophic skin and fusion of the labia) who has been treated over the years with a variety of topical preparations. She has, in addition, a perianal eczematous rash. (b) The patch test results: fragrance is found in many topical preparations and also hygiene sprays and douches. There was a history of using Anusol (containing Balsam of Peru) and Tri-Adcortyl (containing ethylenediamine). Other common allergens implicated in perianal dermatitis are neomycin and benzocaine.

cause of contact dermatitis in this area is rubber. Vaginitis, vulvitis and dermatitis of the penis can be caused by condoms and diaphragms in thiuram/mercaptobenzothiazole (MBT)-sensitive individuals.

VARICOSE ECZEMA

Varicose eczema is the result of venous hypertension in the legs and typically presents as eczema in the gaiter area (Fig 14.7). Associated features include pigmentation (caused by haemosiderin deposition), oedema, lipodermatosclerosis and ulceration. Allergic contact dermatitis is common in patients with stasis eczema and leg ulcers. This is probably the result of a combination of factors, including the chronicity of the condition,

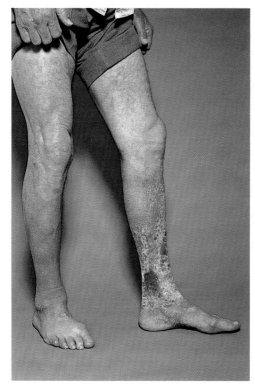

Fig 14.7
Varicose eczema.

and topical preparations being applied to broken skin and often under occlusive bandages. Common causes of allergic contact dermatitis in stasis eczema/leg ulcer patients are shown in Table 14.6.

Management

The key to the long-term management of varicose eczema/venous leg ulcers is compression. If the pedal pulses are difficult to feel, Doppler studies should be undertaken before compression stockings or bandages are fitted. In Doppler studies, the blood pressure is measured in the arm and leg and, if the ratio of arm/leg pressure is > 0.8, support stockings or bandages may be fitted. Support stockings should be put on before

Table 14.6 Common allergens in varicose eczema, with their source and some alternative treatments.

Allergen	Source	Management
Rubber allergens (Thiurams/MBT)	Elastic products	Wear bandages/stockings that do not contain the rubber accelerators (e.g. Setopress and Tensopress)
	Rubber gloves on nurses dressing the legs	Wear vinyl/plastic gloves
Wool alcohols	Creams, e.g. moisturisers, Synalar and Fucidin ointments and Coltapaste bandages, Fucidin Intertulle and Sofra-Tulle	Avoid
Parabens (hydroxybenzoates)	Creams, e.g. moisturisers, Locoid cream and occlusive bandages, e.g. Viscopaste, Quinaband, Tarband, Icthaband	Avoid. Steripaste and Ichthopaste do not contain parabens
Antibiotics/antiseptics, neomycin	Neomycin cream, e.g. Cicatrin Dermovate-NN and Betnovate-N	In general topical antimicrobial preparations should be avoided in these patients
Clioquinol, mupirocin, Betadine	e.g. in Betnovate-C, Bactroban	

MBT, mercaptobenzothiazole.

the patient gets out of bed in the morning and worn throughout the day. The eczema is treated with emollients and topical steroid ointments, e.g. Eumovate (clobetasone butyrate) or Betnovate (betamethasone 0.1%), in association with the compression. More severe cases may need occlusive bandaging with, for example, Steripaste or Ichthopaste.

In view of the high incidence of contact allergy in varicose eczema there should be a low threshold for patch testing. Rubber allergy (to thiuram mix and MBT) is increasing with 15% of leg ulcer/stasis eczema patients having positive patch tests to rubber in a recent study (see Fig 14.8). One reason for this may be the increase in the number of nurses wearing rubber gloves

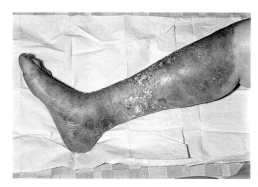

Fig 14.8
Thiuram-allergic patient with
varicose eczema who has
had compression using an
elasticated stocking. Note
the sharp cut-off below
the knee.

Table 14.7 Bandages and stockings that are or are not safe for rubber-allergic patients.

Safe	Not safe
Tensopress	Elastic products
Setopress	Litepress (used in four-layer bandaging)
Comprilan ⎱ Cotton weave Rosidal K ⎰	
Elastane, Lycra and nylon, e.g. Duo-med stockings	

when doing dressings. To avoid this potential source of sensitization, it is
advisable for nurses to wear vinyl or plastic gloves. Table 14.7 shows the
bandages and support stockings that are and are not safe in rubber-allergic
patients.

15 Clinical Features of Contact Dermatitis Caused by Common Allergens

Contact dermatitis can occur at any site depending on the allergen and its source. In this chapter, the common clinical presentations of contact dermatitis caused by the allergens in the Standard European Series (see page 96) are outlined.

NICKEL

Nickel is the most common allergen on patch-testing, with up to 30% of women tested showing positive reactions. Figure 15.1 shows common sources of nickel. The primary site of dermatitis in a nickel-allergic individual occurs at the site of direct contact. In addition, there may be secondary sites involved that are not in direct contact with nickel, resulting in a symmetrical, possibly generalized eruption.

Nickel allergy is up to six times more common in women and sensitization most commonly follows ear piercing, which results in dermatitis over the ear lobes. Most patients with a positive nickel patch test will give a history of reacting to non-silver and non-gold earrings. Even 9- and 18-carat gold can contain small amounts of nickel, which can be significant for some patients. The European Union Directive on Nickel stated that, from 1996, all jewellery must contain less than 0.05% nickel and release less than 0.5 $\mu g/cm^2$ per week. It is hoped that as this takes effect the huge increase in nickel allergy seen over the past 20 years will start to decline.

Figure 15.2 shows the typical periumbilical dermatitis caused by the nickel in stud buttons, in particular those found in jeans. Patients find that covering the stud with nail varnish or material may prevent the dermatitis; however, this often gives only partial or temporary relief. Replacing the stud with a nickel-free alternative, e.g. stainless steel, plastic or brass, is the best

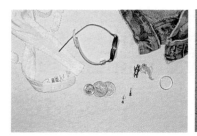
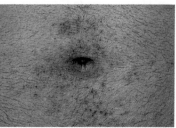

Fig 15.1 Common sources of nickel: jewellery, watches, coins, jeans studs, bra fasteners.

Fig 15.2 Periumbilical dermatitis caused by a jeans stud in a nickel-allergic patient.

solution. Contact with nickel-containing coins generally does not produce a dermatitis unless it is prolonged, e.g. in a cashier.

It has been suggested that dietary nickel can occasionally exacerbate hand dermatitis in a nickel-sensitive individual. Exacerbation of hand dermatitis after oral challenge with nickel and improvement of dermatitis in patients on a nickel-free diet have been demonstrated. However, even in these patients this is seldom useful in practice because of the difficulty of eliminating nickel from the diet.

COBALT

A positive patch test result to cobalt usually occurs in association with a positive test result to nickel, probably because the two metals frequently coexist. Cobalt allergy has also been reported in association with paints, varnishes and cement.

CHROMATE

The most common causes of chromate allergy are cement and chrome-tanned leather. Chromate allergy commonly presents as a hand dermatitis in builders and as foot dermatitis in those allergic to leather. The foot dermatitis tends to be symmetrical, affecting the dorsum (Fig 15.3). Chromate-allergic patients who wear leather shoes develop dermatitis despite wearing socks. Those with foot dermatitis are committed to wearing either vegetable-tanned leather or leather-free shoes for life. Clarks

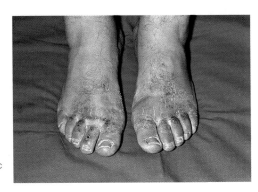

Fig 15.3
Symmetrical acute dermatitis caused by shoe leather in a chromate-allergic patient.

and the Natural Shoe Shop both do a range of vegetable-tanned leather and leather-free shoes (see Appendix). Chromate allergy has a poor prognosis with only around 10% of patients being free of dermatitis after 5 years (see page 76).

FRAGRANCE

Fragrances have widespread uses and are found in cosmetics, hair and skin products, detergents, air fresheners, etc. Fragrance allergy usually results in dermatitis but photodermatitis, urticaria and depigmentation may also be seen. Allergy to fragrances is second to nickel as a cause of a positive patch test. Patients are patch tested to a mixture of eight different fragrances—fragrance mix: cinnamic aldehyde, cinnamic alcohol, eugenol, amylcinnamaldehyde, hydroxycitronella, geraniol, isoeugenol and oakmoss absolute, with sorbitan sesquioleate as emulsifier. All cosmetics are labelled with their ingredients using the INCI nomenclature (see page 70). Fragranced substances are labelled 'parfum'.

Balsam of Peru

Balsam of Peru (INCI name myroxyion pereirae) is tested separately and is a naturally occurring fragrance, obtained from trees, composed of several allergens. Of cases of fragrance mix allergy, 50% also react to Balsam of Peru.

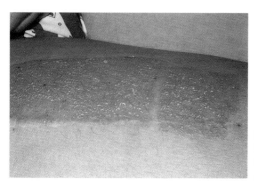

Fig 15.4
Eczematous reaction
to sticking plaster in a
colophony-allergic patient.

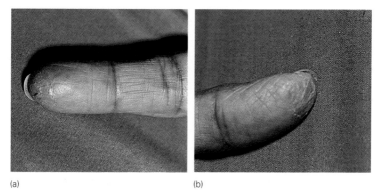

(a)   (b)

Fig 15.5 (a) Chronic dermatitis of (a) the index finger and (b) the thumb of an office worker allergic to colophony.

Colophony

Colophony (INCI name colophonium) is a naturally occurring substance derived from trees. Common sources of colophony include sticking plasters (Fig 15.4) and glues, wax depilatories and some paper. Figure 15.5 shows dermatitis on the index finger and thumb caused by colophony allergy in an office worker.

RUBBER

Raw rubber is not elastic but vulcanization makes the rubber stretchable. Several accelerators used to speed up this process are potent sensitizers.

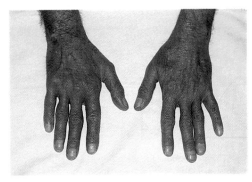

Fig 15.6
Symmetrical hand dermatitis caused by rubber gloves in a patient allergic to thiurams. This patient had some atrophic changes resulting from prolonged steroid use.

The common accelerators that are included in the standard battery are *N*-isopropyl-*N*-phenyl-4-phenylenediamine (IPPD) (found in heavy-duty rubber, e.g. tyres) and mercaptobenzothiazole (MBT) and two mixes of allergens—namely, thiuram and mercapto mix. Rubber gloves are the most common cause, with thiurams being the most frequent allergen. This classically presents with a hand dermatitis that extends up the mid-forearm (Fig 15.6). Patients with a rubber allergy should avoid rubber gloves and wear PVC plastic gloves, or 'hypoallergenic' rubber gloves (which have been washed many times to remove accelerators).

Rubber allergy may also present as foot dermatitis. This typically affects the sole of the foot and plantar aspect of the toes, with sparing of the instep. It may be caused by the rubber in the sole of the shoe or insole. Other sources of rubber that may result in allergic reactions include condoms, rubber in the elastic of underwear and clothes, and elasticated bandages, particularly in leg ulcer/stasis dermatitis patients.

DYES

P-Phenylenediamine (PPD) is a colourless compound that acts as a primary intermediate in permanent hair dyes and clothing dyes. Allergy to dyes may have a variety of presentations. In hairdressers, it may present with a hand dermatitis (Fig 15.7) and, in individuals who use permanent hair dyes, it can result in an eczematous reaction not only on the scalp but also along the hairline (Fig 15.8). An allergy to dyes in the clothes can give an eczematous reaction, the site depending on the clothes involved. Tights are relatively

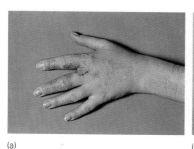
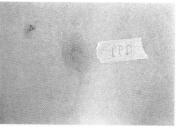

(a)   (b)

Fig 15.7 (a) Hand dermatitis in a hairdresser allergic to *p*-phenylenediamine (PPD).
(b) The patient's positive patch test result.

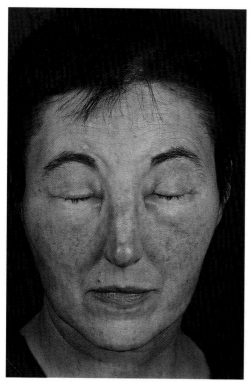

Fig 15.8
Acute allergic reaction to
PPD in permanent hair dye.
Note the dermatitis around
the hairline and orbital
oedema.

common causes of dye-induced clothing dermatitis. Allergy to dyes in tops typically affects the anterior folds of the axilla, with sparing of the apex of the axilla. Patients with a clothing dye dermatitis are advised to avoid wearing dark clothing against the skin and to wear natural materials (e.g. cotton and wool) because these are less likely to release dyes compared with synthetic materials.

4-*tert*-BUTYLPHENOL FORMALDEHYDE RESIN (PTBP RESIN)

This is a resin used in adhesives, particularly for sticking leather goods, e.g. shoes and watchstraps. Contact allergy may present as a foot dermatitis (Fig 15.9) or dermatitis at the site of the watchstrap.

EPOXY RESIN

Epoxy resins are sensitizers in their unhardened state and are hardened by adding other compounds. They are used in industry as adhesives, in surface coatings, plastics, paints, etc. In the home situation, 'two-part' glues are the most common cause of epoxy resin allergy.

WOOL ALCOHOLS (LANOLIN ALCOHOLS)

Lanolin is a natural product derived from sheep fleece, composed of alcohols, esters and fatty acids. Wool alcohols are used in topical medicaments and cosmetics. Sensitivity to lanolin is low in normal skin, higher in eczematous skin, and most prevalent in patients with stasis eczema and leg ulcers. Studies have shown that around 13% of leg dermatitis patients were allergic to wool alcohols, and conversely around 70% of patients allergic to a lanolin-containing cream had stasis eczema. Dermatological products that contain wool alcohols include some bath oils (e.g. Oilatum fragrance-free bath additive), emollients, steroid preparations (e.g. Synalar ointment and Hydrocortisyl ointment) and other products, e.g. Fucidin ointment, Coltapaste bandages and Sofra-Tulle. These products must be avoided in wool alcohol-sensitive patients. Wool alcohols may also be found in cosmetics and Amerchol, a lanolin derivative, which is used as an emulsifier and emollient in cosmetic products. The British National Formulary (BNF) states when products contain wool fat and related substances, including lanolin.

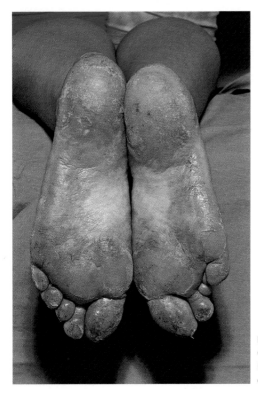

Fig 15.9
Contact dermatitis caused by
PTBP resin. Note the sparing
of the instep.

PRIMIN

Primin is the main allergen in primula dermatitis, which is usually caused by
Primula obconica (Fig 15.10). Primula dermatitis (Fig 15.11) typically
presents as linear streaks on exposed sites and often the clinical diagnosis
is not suspected.

SESQUITERPENE LACTONE MIX

Sesquiterpene lactones are contact allergens present in the Compositae
species. These include weeds (e.g. tansy, milfoil and wild camomile),
flowers (e.g. chrysanthemums and marigolds) and edible plants (e.g.
lettuce, endive and artichoke). Many of the Compositae species are known

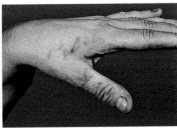

Fig 15.11 Streaky dermatitis in a primin-allergic patient.

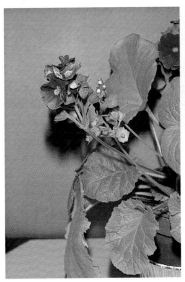

Fig 15.10 *Primula obconica*: the allergen is in the leaves and is released with gentle touching.

to cause an allergic contact dermatitis. This may be localized to the site of contact or be an airborne dermatitis (Fig 15.12) and often there is a history of summer exacerbation of the dermatitis.

PRESERVATIVES

Preservatives found in the standard battery are formaldehyde, parabens mix (methyl-4-hydroxybenzoate, ethyl-4-hydroxybenzoate, propyl-4-hydroxybenzoate, butyl-4-hydroxybenzoate) and quaternium 15.

Formaldehyde

Formaldehyde is present in many different types of products and is a potent sensitizer in industry, hospitals and the home. It is used as a preservative in skin and hair care products, deodorants, washing-up liquid, etc. It is also found in paints, dry cleaning materials, wart treatments, photographic developing materials, paper industry and embalming solutions.

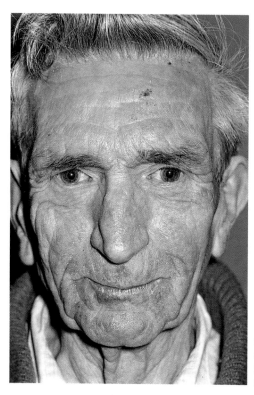

Fig 15.12
Chronic facial dermatitis
in a gardener allergic to
sesquiterpene lactone.

Formaldehyde dermatitis from fabrics is less commonly seen now because
of improvements in manufacturing, but it may still be found in some crease-
resistant fabrics.

Parabens (hydroxybenzoates)

Parabens are commonly used preservatives found in foods, drugs,
topical medicaments and cosmetics. Although they are widely used in
cosmetics, sensitization is rare in people with healthy skin and is most
commonly seen in patients with stasis eczema, leg ulcers and dermatitis.
In topical medications, they are listed as hydroxybenzoates and are found
in some emollients, topical steroid creams (e.g. Locoid) and lotions, ENT

preparations and occlusive bandages (e.g. Viscopaste, Icthaband, Quinaband, Tarband). Steripaste and Ichthopaste do **not** contain parabens. The BNF states when moisturizers or topical steroids contain hydroxybenzoates.

Many different types of cosmetics may contain parabens, including lipsticks, deodorants, depilatory creams, etc. In keeping with the International Nomenclature for Cosmetic Ingredients (INCI) (see page 70), parabens-containing cosmetics are labelled methylparaben, propylparaben, butylparaben, ethylparaben or benzylparaben, depending on which paraben is present.

Quaternium 15
Quaternium 15 is a formaldehyde releaser used mainly as a preservative in cosmetics, and allergy to this most commonly presents as a facial dermatitis.

Methylchloroisothiazolinone/methylisothiazolinone
This biocide is used as a preservative in cosmetics and is also known as Kathon CG or Cl- + Me-isothiazolinone. However, the full name above is used in the labelling of cosmetics. This biocide is also found in soaps, detergents, shampoos and moist lavatory paper, as well as having some industrial sources.

MEDICAMENTS

Neomycin
This broad-spectrum antibiotic is found in various topical preparations—creams and ointments, powders, ear drops and nose drops. Neomycin usually cross-reacts with other antibiotics in this class, in particular framycetin.

Benzocaine
Benzocaine is a topical local anaesthetic found in haemorrhoid creams, sore throat sprays, burn remedies, etc. Although the official European Standard Battery includes benzocaine, many dermatology departments prefer to patch test to a mixture of benzocaine with other related compounds (Caine

mix) because this increases the identification of individuals with topical local anaesthetic allergy. Lidocaine (lignocaine), which is commonly used as a local anaesthetic in skin surgery and dentistry, is structurally different and safe to use in a benzocaine-allergic individual.

Quinoline mix (clioquinol and chlorquinaldol)

Clioquinol (also known as Vioform) is an anti-infective agent used in topical preparations, e.g. Vioform-Hydrocortisone and Betnovate-C. Chlorquinaldol has similar properties to clioquinol and is also used in some proprietary preparations.

Tixocortol pivalate

Allergy to topical steroids should be suspected in patients whose dermatitis is not responding to, or is being aggravated by, their topical steroids. Tixocortol pivalate is a marker for hydrocortisone allergy and is the most common of the causes of steroid allergy, with positive reactions occurring in up to 4% of patients. Allergy to other topical steroids may also be revealed by a positive reaction to tixocortol pivalate, and adding budesonide to the standard battery increases this pick-up rate.

16 Patch Testing

Patch testing is the procedure used to diagnose contact dermatitis. It involves putting small amounts of diluted potential allergens on the skin and leaving these for 2 days. If a patient is allergic to one of these substances, within this 2-day period a delayed type of hypersensitivity (type IV allergic reaction) will be mounted by the patient, who will then develop an area of dermatitis at the site of the allergen. The concentration of allergen is standardized in order to make it strong enough to produce an allergic reaction in a sensitized individual, but not so strong as to produce an irritant effect. Pre-prepared kits are now available and, although these are more convenient to use and the concentration of allergen more consistent, the number of allergens available for testing is limited. Therefore, many departments prepare their own batteries.

Figure 16.1 shows the equipment needed for patch testing. Most allergens are dissolved in white petroleum; liquid allergens are added to filter paper. A small amount of the allergen is placed in an aluminium disc called a Finn chamber, which is then applied to the upper back. If the patient's back is hairy, shaving may be necessary, although this can result in irritation and make interpretation of the results difficult. The Finn chambers are applied to the back using hypoallergenic tape, which provides occlusion of the Finn chambers; this is important because it reduces the risk of false-negative reactions. If the patient expects to experience hot or humid conditions while having the patch testing, it is advisable to tape the edges of the patches.

The upper back is the ideal site for patch testing. However, if this is not possible, e.g. as a result of dermatitis on the back, the front or limbs may be used. The patches are applied with pressure from the bottom edge up to remove any air pouches. The site of the patches is marked and the patches numbered using a marking pen (Fig 16.2). The patches are removed and first read after 2 days (see page 95 for interpretation of results). A reading plate (see Fig 16.1) with holes at the site of the Finn chambers helps interpretation. The second reading after 4 days is essential. Reactions present on day 2 but gone by day 4 would suggest an irritant effect. The

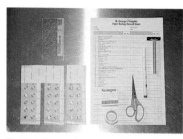

Fig 16.1 The equipment used for patch testing.

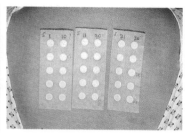

Fig 16.2 The standard battery applied to the back.

results are marked on a prepared sheet as shown in Fig 16.1. This has the standard battery printed on it, and all patients will be tested to this battery. Below this are spaces to add the further batteries that may be tested. The results from day 2 and day 4 are noted.

INFORMATION FOR PATIENTS

When patients attend for patch testing, they are given an information sheet to explain the procedure and how to care for the patch tests (Table 16.1). Patch testing may be carried out at any age, and indeed contact dermatitis in children is being reported more and more. On the whole, pregnant women are not patch tested because, although there is no evidence that

---

How to care for patch tests

Wear an old T-shirt on your first visit to keep the patches in place and avoid staining of clothes

Keep the patches dry—shallow baths only

Avoid exercise that involves excessive arm movement or sweating—this can cause the patches to come off

If the patches become loose, use non-allergic tape (e.g. Micropore) to stick the edges down

Avoid sunbeds or sunbathing (this should also be avoided for 2 weeks before the tests are done)

Table 16.1
Information for patients.

it is harmful, any coincidental miscarriage or fetal malformation may subsequently be blamed on the procedure.

ABOUT PATCH TESTING

Patch testing is designed to see whether a patient is allergic to substances in contact with his or her skin, and is **not** testing foods, dust or pollens. The test involves three visits over 4 days. On the first visit, the patches will be applied to the back; they will be removed on the second visit and, on the final visit, the doctor will discuss the results with the patient (see Table 16.1).

ALLERGEN TESTING

All patients are tested to a standard battery; the European Standard Battery consists of 23 allergens (Table 16.2). However, some dermatology departments add further allergens to give an extended standard battery. In addition, other allergens will be tested depending on the site of the dermatitis, e.g. using facial, shoe, leg ulcer, hairdressing batteries, etc. Patients are asked to bring with them substances to which they think they might be allergic, e.g. cosmetics, creams, shoes, etc. The patient may then be patch tested to these either 'as is' or in the diluted form if necessary.

READING THE RESULTS

Patches should remain in place and are read 2 days later, 15–30 minutes after removing the patches. The second reading is best done on day 4. At the second reading, one can see which reactions have disappeared (suggesting an irritant reaction on day 2) and which have appeared or increased in intensity (suggesting allergy).

The results of patch tests are recorded using a grading system recommended by the International Contact Dermatitis Research Group (Table 16.3).

Irritant reactions tend to be sore compared with allergic reactions which are often itchy. Irritant reactions do not extend beyond the area covered by the Finn chamber and are characterized by such changes as fine wrinkling, petechiae, bullae or necrosis. Although the patch test results are graded as shown in Table 16.3, in practical terms the advice given to patients is the same whether they have had a '+' or '+++' reaction, i.e. they are allergic to

Table 16.2 The European Standard Battery.

Allergen	Common source
Potassium dichromate	Leather, e.g. shoes
P-phenylenediamine base	Hair dye
Rubber accelerators, e.g. thiuram mix	Rubber products, e.g. rubber gloves
Neomycin	Creams
Nickel and cobalt	Non-silver/non-gold jewellery
Benzocaine	Topical local anaesthetic preparations
Quinoline mix	Topical anti-infection creams
Colophony	Sticking plasters
Parabens	Preservative in creams, cosmetics, etc.
Wool alcohols (lanolin)	Ointment base in cosmetics and creams
Epoxy resin	In adhesives
Myroxylon pereirae (Balsam of Peru)	Fragrance in foods and topical preparations
4-*tert*-Butylphenol formaldehyde resin	Glues, e.g. for sticking leather
Formaldehyde	Preservative in cosmetics, shampoos, etc.
Fragrance mix	In fragranced substances
Sesquiterpone lactone mix	Marker for allergy to Compositae
Quaternium 15	Preservative, e.g. in cosmetics
Primin	Marker for primula allergy
Chloro-methyl-isothiazolinone	Preservative in cosmetics, shampoos, creams, etc.

the substance tested. Figure 16.3a shows a '++' allergic reaction to nickel; Fig 16.3b shows a bullous irritant reaction to mascara. Mascara should not be used for patch testing as it can be irritant when applied under occlusion.

A positive reaction may be particularly difficult to interpret when testing the patient's products because the concentration is not standardized. The substance can be tested at different concentrations—an irritant reaction should show a clear increase in the severity of the reaction with increasing

Table 16.3 Grading system for patch test results of International Contact Dermatitis Research Group.

?+	Doubtful reaction: faint erythema only
+	Weak positive reaction: erythema, infiltration, possibly papules
++	Strong positive reaction: erythema, infiltration, papules, vesicles
+++	Extreme positive reaction: intense erythema and infiltration and coalescing vesicles
IR	Irritant reaction
NT	Not tested

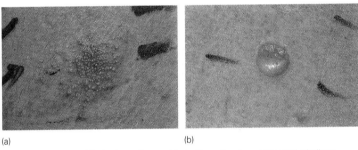

(a)   (b)

Fig 16.3 This shows (a) a '++' reaction to nickel with coalescing vesicles; (b) a bullous irritant reaction after patch testing to mascara.

concentration. Alternatively, the substance can be tested on controls and, if the same concentration fails to produce a reaction in controls, it is likely that the patient's reaction is an allergic one.

DISCUSSING THE RESULTS WITH THE PATIENT

Once patch tests have been read, the patient is informed of the results. The dermatologist will go through the results with the patient to try to ascertain which results are relevant to the dermatitis. The dermatologist should go through an information sheet given to the patient, which outlines preparations containing the allergen so the patient can consider sources of exposure. It is essential to explain to patients that allergic reactions are life-long and that therefore the allergens will always need to be avoided.

If the relevance of a result is in doubt, a repeat open application test (ROAT) may be carried out. The patient is asked to apply the substance twice a day to the same spot on the volar aspect of the forearm for up to a week. If an area of dermatitis develops at this site after 2–4 days, it is likely that this is an allergic reaction.

Key points

1   Patch testing is the test used to diagnose contact dermatitis.

2   Subirritant concentrations of substances are applied to the skin under occlusion. The results are read on days 2 and 4.

3   Irritant reactions tend to improve by day 4, whereas allergic ones become more pronounced. Although irritant reactions tend to have different morphology compared with allergic ones, they can be difficult to distinguish.

4   The results need to be explained to the patient who should be aware that the allergies are generally life-long.

17 Contact Urticaria and the Role of Other Allergy Tests

Unlike contact dermatitis, which is a delayed-type hypersensitivity reaction and is diagnosed using patch testing, contact urticaria is an acute reaction that may be divided into non-immunological and immunological (allergic).

TESTS USED IN NON-IMMUNOLOGICAL AND IMMUNOLOGICAL URTICARIA

Non-immunological contact urticaria

To test for non-immunological urticaria, a small amount of the substance is placed on the flexure surface of the forearm and the results recorded after 45 minutes. Patients should not have taken non-steroidal anti-inflammatories or antihistamines for 2 days before the test. The results may be dose dependent, with erythema and itching occurring at lower concentrations and urticaria developing at higher strengths. The sensitivity of different sites is variable, the face being more sensitive than the limbs, and contact urticaria may explain why some patients develop irritancy to facial creams but patch tests are negative.

Allergic contact urticaria

There are various methods for testing immediate hypersensitivity as shown in Table 17.1.

Table 17.1
Tests for immediate hypersensitivity.

Open application test
Skin-prick test
Prick-prick test
Scratch test

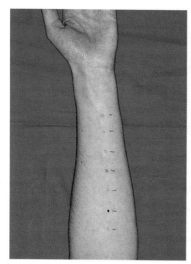

Fig 17.1 The different allergens to be tested are placed on the forearm.

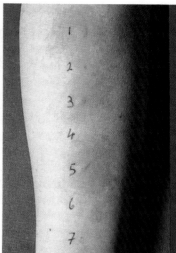

Fig 17.2 Prick tests showing positive reaction.

There is a small risk of anaphylaxis when testing patients with allergic contact urticaria, and it should be done only in a clinical setting with a doctor and resuscitation facilities available.

Open application test

The substance to be tested is placed on the forearm on an area approximately 1 × 1 cm. Redness or a weal after 15 minutes indicates a positive reaction.

Skin-prick tests

There are a large number of commercial allergen solutions now available. Small drops of the solutions to be tested are placed well spaced out on the volar aspect of the forearm, along with histamine as a positive and saline as a negative control (Fig 17.1). Using a special lancet, the epidermis is gently raised. After 15 minutes, the results are read and reactions that are 3 mm larger than the controls are considered positive (Fig 17.2).

Prick-prick test and scratch test

These methods are used if standardized allergens are not available. In the prick-prick test the substance to be tested, e.g. food, is pricked and the lancet then used as in a skin-prick test (see Fig 17.4). In the scratch test a 0.5-cm scratch is made on the forearm (without drawing blood) and a small amount of the allergen is placed on the scratch. In both cases, histamine is used as a positive and saline as a negative control, and results equal to or greater than the histamine reaction after 15 minutes are considered to be positive.

CAUSES OF CONTACT URTICARIA

Non-immunological contact urticaria

Non-immunological contact urticaria occurs without previous sensitization in most exposed individuals. It is less potentially serious than the allergic type because severe systemic reactions are not produced. Examples of substances producing this type of urticaria are shown in Table 17.2.

Allergic contact urticaria

Allergic contact urticaria is an immediate type I hypersensitivity occurring in sensitized individuals; it is more common in atopic individuals and is mediated by the immunoglobulin IgE. Examples of substances producing this type of urticaria are shown in Table 17.3.

Table 17.2 Examples of substances causing non-immunological contact urticaria and potential sources.

Cause of non-immunological contact urticaria	Source
Sorbic acid, benzoic acid, cinnamic acid, cinnamic aldehyde	Preservatives, fragrances and flavourings in foods, soaps, mouthwashes, topical agents, etc.
Stinging nettles	
Jelly fish	

Table 17.3 Examples of substances causing allergic contact urticaria and potential sources.

Cause of immunological (allergic) reactions	Source
Latex	Rubber
Foods, e.g. egg, milk, potato, meat, fish, fruits and nuts	
Topical drugs, e.g. penicillin, neomycin, bacitracin, benzocaine	
Saliva	Dog
Seminal fluid	Human seminal fluid

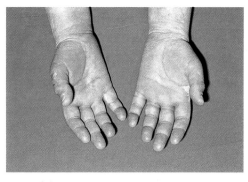

Fig 17.3
Acute urticaria from rubber gloves in a latex-sensitive patient.

Latex allergy

The best known cause of allergic contact urticaria is latex allergy. The tree *Hevea brasiliensis* produces natural rubber latex and the allergens are in the protein fraction. The rising use of rubber gloves in the hospital setting over the past 10 years has been associated with an increase in latex allergy. This has been partly attributed to the use of poorer quality rubber gloves, which release the latex proteins more readily. Of latex allergic patients, 80% are atopic, and groups at high risk include health-care workers, patients who have had multiple operations (particularly abdominal operations) and spina bifida patients. Patients describe itching, wealing and swelling (Fig 17.3) within minutes to an hour after contact. Airborne latex particles (which are particularly prevalent with powdered latex gloves) may result in rhinitis, conjunctivitis and wheezing. Anaphylaxis may occur in any sensitized individual, but is most common when the latex contact is mucosal,

Table 17.4 Common sources of rubber latex and non-latex alternatives.

Contains latex	Safe alternative
Rubber gloves	Wear PVC/plastic gloves
Balloons	
Rubber tubing used in hospital procedures	Latex-free tubing is available
Barrier contraceptives	Avanti condoms

e.g. during abdominal operations, vaginal and dental examinations, etc. Common sources of latex-containing entities are shown in Table 17.4.

In addition, certain foods may cross-react with latex, e.g. chestnuts, avocados, bananas, peaches and passion fruit, and these should be avoided in latex-allergic individuals.

Diagnosis of latex allergy

If there is a history of anaphylaxis, challenging to latex must be avoided and a radioallergosorbent test (RAST) to latex should be done. The RAST measures the amount of latex-specific IgE in the patient's serum. It is important when doing RASTs that the total IgE is also measured, because a borderline-positive RAST is less likely to be significant in association with a very high IgE. If there is no contraindication, the patient should be tested to a glove, initially using a finger-stall and, if this produces no reaction, then using the whole glove. The development of urticaria confirms an allergy to latex. If this does not produce a reaction, prick testing to latex solution (using histamine as a positive and physiological saline as a negative control) may be carried out.

Management of latex allergy

Health-care workers should wear vinyl or plastic gloves where possible. Latex-free sterile rubber gloves are available (e.g. Allergard [Johnson & Johnson]) and these should be ordered as necessary. Patients must be aware of what contains latex and should avoid it, and in particular inform dentists and doctors if they are to have a surgical procedure. Many hospital trusts have banned the use of powdered latex gloves in an attempt to reduce the rising incidence of latex allergy in health-care workers.

FOODS

Foods are the most common cause of immediate hypersensitivity reaction. The orolaryngeal area is usually affected. This may result in swelling of the lips, tongue and throat. Anaphylaxis is the extreme response seen with some foods, most commonly nuts.

Nut allergy

The incidence of nut allergy has increased in the past few years, and food manufacturers are becoming increasingly aware of the problem; many of them are labelling products that contain nuts. It is not entirely clear why there has been this increase in nut allergy. In view of the fact that nut allergy is much more common in atopic individuals, it is recommended that atopic children avoid nuts until the age of 4 years.

If there is a history of a severe reaction, RASTs should be used to diagnose nut allergy. If not, prick tests may be carried out using commercial solutions. Often patients are allergic to more than one nut type, peanuts being the most common. It is recommended that nut-allergic patients avoid all nuts, however, because contamination by different nuts is possible. Most childhood nut allergies continue into adult life. Patients with severe nut allergy should carry epinephrine (adrenaline) in the form of an Epipen in case of inadvertent exposure.

Eggs and milk

Contact urticaria to milk and eggs is common in atopic infants, but most children grow out of these allergies by the age of 5 years. Skin contact with eggs or milk results in urticaria and ingestion may be accompanied by lip swelling, widespread erythema, urticaria, vomiting and wheezing. Children can be intermittently tested in a hospital setting by an open application test, first to the arm and, if there is no reaction, the mucosal surface of the lip. If these reactions are negative, oral challenge or prick tests may be done.

Contact urticaria in food handlers

Contact urticaria in food handlers is most commonly seen in patients with hand dermatitis (Fig 17.4). Patients describe immediate itching and weal formation on touching certain foods. Common offenders are raw potatoes, fish, meat (usually a specific meat), tomatoes and fruits. Eating the foods is

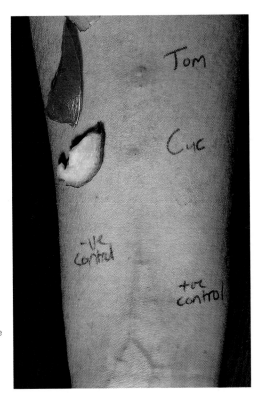

Fig 17.4
This school dinner lady had hand dermatitis, which was very much worse in term time, with stinging and itching when she touched certain foods. The photograph shows a positive prick-prick test to tomato and cucumber; histamine-positive and saline-negative controls are also shown.

generally safe and it is likely that cooking and the action of digestion renders the foods 'hypoallergenic' for the patient. Patients should be tested using the prick-prick test or scratch test and, once the diagnosis is established, wear gloves to avoid contact with the foods.

18 When are Allergy Tests Inappropriate?

Dermatologists frequently have patients referred to them who have chronic generalized urticaria or atopic dermatitis, where the patient has requested 'allergy testing'. Patients' perception of allergy testing generally refers to prick and radioallergosorbent tests (RASTs) as opposed to patch testing.

CHRONIC GENERALIZED URTICARIA

Over 90% of patients with urticaria referred to a dermatologist will have idiopathic chronic urticaria. In this condition, bouts of weals develop, sometimes daily, and the episodes last longer than 6 weeks (Fig 18.1). Patch testing has no role in this condition and tests of immediate hypersensitivity are generally unhelpful. Patients should be advised to avoid known precipitants of urticaria (e.g. excess caffeine, aspirin, non-steroidal anti-inflammatory drugs (NSAIDs), etc.) and treated with a non-sedative antihistamine, e.g. loratadine (Clarityn), fexofenadine hydrochloride (Telfast 180) or cetirizine (Zirtek).

Acute generalized urticaria lasts only a few days. Often no cause is found, but it may be attributed to a certain food (where RAST or prick testing would be appropriate), drug or viral infection.

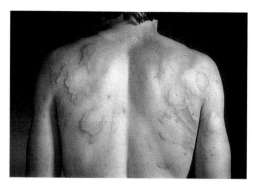

Fig 18.1
Patient with chronic urticaria showing the typical weals and wealing at the site of scratching (dermatographism).

ATOPIC DERMATITIS

Parents of children with atopic dermatitis and adult patients are often very keen to know about potential allergens, in particular allergens in foods. Assessing dietary precipitants can be difficult because the natural course in atopic dermatitis is to remit and flare. Infants with cows' milk sensitivity may present with widespread dermatitis which improves with avoidance of cows' milk formula (substituting with soya milk or a milk hydrolysate, e.g. Nutramigen). In children with severe dermatitis, dietary restriction can result in an improvement in their dermatitis (see page 16). It is important that this is undertaken in a controlled fashion with a dietitian to ensure adequate nutrition. Allergy testing (i.e. RAST and prick testing) is not, however, a reliable way of detecting which foods it would be helpful to exclude. Prick testing in atopic dermatitis is neither sensitive nor specific and the results show a poor correlation with the clinical improvement seen with dietary restriction. In adult patients dietary restriction is, in general, unhelpful. However, if there is a recrudescence of atopic dermatitis after many years of remission, patch testing should be considered (see page 66). Table 18.1 summarizes when to use allergy tests.

Table 18.1 When to allergy test.

Condition	Type of test	
	Prick/RAST/prick-prick etc.	Patch test
Atopic dermatitis—children	No	Occasionally
Atopic dermatitis—adults	No	Sometimes
Acute urticaria	Yes	Sometimes
Chronic urticaria	No	No
Contact urticaria	Yes	No
Contact dermatitis	No	Yes

Appendix

LEATHER-FREE SHOES
Clarks International
PO Box 4
Street
Somerset
BA16 0YA
Tel: 01458 443 131

VEGETABLE DYE SHOES
Natural Shoe Store
21 Neal Street
Covent Garden
London
WC2H 9 PU
Tel: 020 7836 5254

Natural Shoe Store
325 King's Road
London
SW3 5ES
Tel: 020 7351 3721

Vegetarian Shoes
12 Gardner Street
Brighton
BN1 1UP
Tel: 01273 691 913

Index